W9-BMA-921

LUMBAR DISC DISEASE

A TWENTY-YEAR CLINICAL FOLLOW-UP STUDY

LUMBAR DISC DISEASE

A TWENTY-YEAR CLINICAL FOLLOW-UP STUDY

Edited by

Blaine S. Nashold, Jr., M.D.

Associate Professor of Neurosurgery, Department of Surgery,
Duke University Medical Center, Durham, N. C.

Zdenek Hrubec, Sc.D.

Statistician, Follow-up Agency, Division of Medical Sciences,
National Research Council, Washington, D. C.

A Cooperative Study of 17 Veterans Administration Hospitals
and the Follow-up Agency, Division of Medical Sciences,
National Research Council

The work reported herein is part of the program of studies of the Follow-up Agency,
Division of Medical Sciences, National Research Council, developed by the
Committee on Veterans Medical Problems in cooperation with the Veterans
Administration and the Department of Defense, and presently conducted under the
direction of the Committee on Epidemiology and Veterans Follow-up Studies.
The investigation was supported by the Veterans Administration contract
number VAm-22734 on the specific advice of the Committee on Veterans
Medical Problems.

THE C. V. MOSBY COMPANY

Saint Louis   1971

Copyright © 1971 by The C. V. Mosby Company

All rights reserved. No part of this book may be reproduced
or utilized in any form or by any means without permission
from the publisher, except for the purpose of official use
by the United States Government.

Printed in the United States of America

International Standard Book Number 0-8016-3625-6

Library of Congress Catalog Card Number 72-174782

Distributed in Great Britain by Henry Kimpton, London

EDITORIAL COMMITTEE

COCHAIRMEN

Blaine S. Nashold, Jr., M.D., *Chairman of study*

Zdenek Hrubec, Sc.D., *Statistician*

MEMBERS

Emanuele Mannarino, M.D.

Chief, Neurosurgical Section, Department of Medicine and Surgery,
Veterans Administration, Washington, D. C.

James E. Nixon, M.D.

Chief, Orthopedic Section, Veterans Hospital, Philadelphia, Pa.

Hubert L. Rosomoff, M.D.

Professor and Chairman, Division of Neurological Surgery,
Miami University School of Medicine, Miami, Fla.

Charles B. Wilson, M.D.

Professor and Chairman, Division of Neurological Surgery,
University of California, San Francisco Medical Center,
San Francisco, Calif.

PARTICIPANTS

Clinical participants—Neurosurgeons

Blaine S. Nashold, Jr., M.D., CHAIRMAN, VAH, *Durham, N. C.*
J. William Blaisdell, M.D., VAH, *San Francisco, Calif.*
August Buermann, M.D., VAH, *Coral Gables, Fla.*
H. M. Dratz, M.D., VAH, *Albany, N. Y.*
William A. Kelly, M.D., VAH, *Seattle, Wash.*
Erich G. Krueger, M.D., VAH, *The Bronx, New York, N. Y.*
R. C. Llewellyn, M.D., VAH, *New Orleans, La.*
Robert W. Porter, M.D., VAH, *Long Beach, Calif.*
Hubert L. Rosomoff, M.D., VAH, *Pittsburgh, Pa.*
Dan Ruge, M.D., VAH (Research), *Chicago, Ill.*
George T. Tindall, M.D., VAH, *Durham, N. C.*
Jack L. Ulmer, M.D., VAH, *Richmond, Va.*
Charles B. Wilson, M.D., University of Kentucky School of Medicine,
  Lexington, Ky.

Clinical participants—Orthopedists

Murray E. Gibbens, M.D., VAH, *Denver, Colo.*
Robert H. Hutchinson, M.D., VAH, *Long Beach, Calif.*
J. F. Kurtz, M.D., VAH, *Hines, Ill.*
James E. Nixon, M.D., VAH, *Philadelphia, Pa.*
Robert F. Premer, M.D., VAH, *Minneapolis, Minn.*
David Schwartz, M.D., VAH, *Albany, N. Y.*
Troy H. Smith, M.D., VAH, *San Francisco, Calif.*
George Truchly, M.D., VAH, *New York, N. Y.*

Clinical participant—Neurologist

Paul B. Jossmann, M.D., VAH, *Boston, Mass.*

Radiologists

Lewis R. Lawrence, M.D., CHAIRMAN, VAH, *New York, N. Y.*
Harry L. Barton, M.D., VAH, *Houston, Tex.*
Johan Bonk, M.D., VAH, *Durham, N. C.*
Benjamin E. Greenberg, M.D., VAH, *Memphis, Tenn.*
Miriam Liberson, M.D., VAH (West Side), *Chicago, Ill.*
Walter H. Mendel, M.D., VAH, *Richmond, Va.*

Charles P. Oderr, M.D., VAH, *New Orleans, La.*
Sidney Traub, M.D., University of Oklahoma, *Oklahoma City, Okla.*
Sol Unger, M.D., VAH, *The Bronx, New York, N. Y.*
Egon Wissing, M.D., VAH, *Boston, Mass.*

Veterans Administration Central Office (VACO)

J. A. Kennedy, M.D., *Washington, D. C.*
Lyndon E. Lee, M.D., *Washington, D. C.*
Emanuele Mannarino, M.D., *Washington, D. C.*
Mark Wolcott, M.D., *Washington, D. C.*

Follow-up Agency, Division of Medical Sciences, National Research Council

Zdenek Hrubec, Sc.D., *Washington, D. C.*
M. Dean Nefzger, Ph.D., *Washington, D. C.*

Consultant

Barnes Woodhall, M.D., Duke University Medical Center, *Durham, N. C.*

FOREWORD

Early in World War II, Dr. R. Glen Spurling, then Major Spurling, assembled a conference of some forty-odd young neurosurgeons who had recently volunteered for Army service. The conference was held at the Walter Reed General Hospital in Washington, D. C., and its avowed purpose was to preview combat and non-combat injuries. Such injuries were, presently, to fill a large number of hospitals in combat areas overseas and in nineteen neurosurgical centers in the United States. It was a rather unusual experience, and for recently recruited Army neurosurgeons, one that will probably not be repeated in the era of the draft.

Major attention was directed toward gunshot wounds of the brain, spinal cord, and peripheral nerves, and at implementing training programs in neurosurgery for young general surgeons. With the campaigns then contemplated, it was clear that experienced neurosurgeons would be in short supply and unable to handle the large numbers of casualties expected. All agreed that a purely military prototype must be constructed. As a minor historic footnote, it should be said that these converted general surgeons did a magnificent job.

There were also some comments about the surgical treatment of sciatica, accurately identified some ten years earlier by Mixter and Barr as a sign of ruptured intervertebral disc. Their findings had been presented before the New England Surgical Society in 1933, and subsequently published in the *New England Journal of Medicine*. No one at that conference even vaguely dreamed, however, that 14,000 cases would be diagnosed during World War II as "herniated nucleus pulposus" or that by 1959 the Veterans Administration would be compensating about 16,000 World War II veterans for herniated nucleus pulposus incurred in, or aggravated by, military service.

Elsewhere in this monograph are described the various advantages and disadvantages of the study as they were postulated in 1958-1959. Two disadvantages might be emphasized. The first is the relative inexperience of most of the military surgeons with this particular problem, with its wide diagnostic and treatment spectra. The second has to do with the changing directives by which Army authorities sought to increase the effectiveness of their manpower or to protect the soldier from undue risk. In many respects this effort to review a wartime injury proved to be more difficult than those concerned with brain or peripheral nerve injuries.

An unexpected appointment as Dean of the Duke University Medical School prevented me from participating in this meticulous enterprise. I am grateful to Dr. Blaine S. Nashold, Jr., for accepting the chairmanship of this cooperative study. All patients with this disturbing syndrome would feel grateful to Dr. Nashold and his many colleagues if they too knew the potential significance of the findings.

BARNES WOODHALL

PREFACE

Long-term follow-up studies such as this one require an expertise and wealth of resource that only a large agency such as the Veterans Administration can mobilize and support. Because of their complexity, these studies are necessarily rare. The wide variety of scientific and clinical talent employed in the design and execution of this investigation has produced definitive data on many aspects of lumbar intervertebral disc disease and the disability associated with it. A major goal of this work—to throw light on the life history of the disease—was only partly realized, and we advanced little in the art of prognosis. As often happens in scientific endeavors, the answers at which we arrive unveil new questions requiring further research. The view of lumbar disc disease that emerges is that of a complex disorder that must be considered in the context of the more comprehensive degenerative back syndrome. The subject will require further long-term studies, including regular periodic assessment of changes and an experimental approach to the evaluation of therapy.

Our report was written not only for the specialist but also for the general practitioner. The summaries at the end of each chapter and the final summary were so organized that they may be used as a guide for the clinical evaluation of the patient with lumbar disc disease. The Appendix will give future investigators the details of methodology and organization of the present study, and the bibliography provides a convenient entry to the literature on this subject. The specialist, whether he be a neurologist, neurosurgeon, orthopedist, radiologist, or epidemiologist, should be able to use the data to broaden and strengthen his own concepts of disc disease. Agencies concerned with health care and its delivery will also find useful this study of a common cause of disability. Finally, we hope that from this work direct benefits will accrue to the patient suffering from the effects of disc disease.

The study owes its origin to the interest and foresight of Dr. Barnes Woodhall, who even during World War II clearly perceived the need for follow-up studies and established in the Army the Peripheral Nerve Registry that provided the basis for his extensive postwar monograph. Dr. Woodhall proposed that intervertebral disc lesions be similarly investigated, and he participated in the early planning that led to the present study.

The study received support at each of the seventeen Veterans Administration (VA) examining centers through the administrator in the form of secretarial and ancillary services. Social service departments of the various examining centers worked with patients to facilitate their participation in the follow-up examination. Mrs. Virginia Karl from the VACO coordinated the activities of the social service departments.

The clinical program started in July 1961 and continued through 1964. Eligible subjects who resided within a reasonable traveling distance from the examining centers were scheduled for a follow-up evaluation, which included neurologic diagnostic procedures and roentgenograms of the lumbar spine. A preliminary analysis was carried out with the assistance of committees of the clinical participants and radiologists.

Members of the Radiology Committee reviewed the roentgenograms of the study, and some of them were instrumental in obtaining the follow-up films. In most of the hospitals the radiology departments contributed their services in obtaining the follow-up roentgenograms without other relationship to the study. Much of the early planning in the area of radiology is due to Dr. Sidney Traub, who was unable to continue with the project in its later phases.

The Medical Statistics Agency, Office of The Surgeon General, U. S. Army, provided the roster from which the sample was compiled. The VA resources made it possible to obtain the addresses of the patients and their medical records, and the General Services Administration National Personnel Records Center made available relevant Army service records with the approval of the Army. The *Journal of the American Medical Association* kindly gave us permission to reproduce material in the Appendix on the measurement of spine motion. Dr. Haymaker, Dr. Woodhall, and The W. B. Saunders Company were generous in agreeing to our use in the Appendix of a chart showing dermatome distribution.

The operations staff of the Follow-up Agency, Division of Medical Sciences, National Academy of Sciences–National Research Council, was directed by Mr. A. Hiram Simon. Records work at the National Personnel Records Center was supervised by Mrs. Dorothy J. Mahon. Mrs. Jeanne Downie supervised allocation of patients for the clinical examinations. The records abstracting staff, under the supervision of Mrs. Vivian Farley, abstracted the service hospital records and coded the medical information essential to the study.

The participation of the Follow-up Agency was funded by the VA through contract number VAm-22734.

BLAINE S. NASHOLD, JR.
ZDENEK HRUBEC

CONTENTS

CHAPTER *1*

HISTORICAL PERSPECTIVE AND BACKGROUND

BLAINE S. NASHOLD, JR.

Intervertebral disc disease, evaluated in terms of its life history, represents one of the most complex medical disorders. When ancestral man traded his arboreal existence for that of an erect biped, the stage may have been set for development of this disorder through the introduction of mechanical stresses on the vertebral structures for which they were not adequately designed. A clinical investigator who studies a disease that may last the lifetime of the patient can expect to observe only part of the total pathologic process. To piece together the entire puzzle will require studies by two or three generations of investigators. This report is an attempt to describe a segment of the life history of men suffering from lumbar disc disease during their Army experience in World War II and to relate it to another cross-sectional view of the same group about 20 years later.

Vesalius[1] described the gross anatomy of the intervertebral disc and differentiated it from the annulus fibrosus. A sketch of a traumatically herniated disc appeared in the anatomic drawings of Charles Bell[2] in 1824. But the modern investigative era began in 1857 with Virchow,[3] and later in 1858 Von Luschka[4] carried out studies on the anatomy and pathology of the intervertebral disc. An early clinical description of a lumbar disc lesion compressing the cauda equina at the L3 level was reported by Krause and Oppenheim[5] in 1909. In 1929 Dandy[6] operated on 2 patients whose preoperative diagnosis was malignant disease of the spinal canal. He removed free fragments of herniated degenerated disc that had compressed the cauda equina, and he commented that "this lesion offers a pathological basis for cases of so-called sciatica, especially bilateral sciatica."

In 1932 Mixter and Barr[7] discussed a patient with severe sciatica resulting from a skiing accident. The initial diagnosis was spinal tumor, but the authors concluded that the diagnosis was more likely enchondroma, and the surgical specimen proved to be a fragment of intervertebral disc. They then reviewed the case

[1]Vesalius, A.: De humani corporis fabrica libri septem, Basileae, 1543, J. Oporinum, pp. 57-59.
[2]Bell, C.: Observations on injuries of the spine and of the thigh bone, London, 1824, Thomas Tegg.
[3]Virchow, R.: Untersuchungen über die Entwicklung des Schadelgrundes, Berlin, 1857, George Reimer.
[4]Von Luschka, H.: Die Halgelenke des neuschlichen Korpers, Berlin, 1858, George Reimer.
[5]Krause, F., and Oppenheim, H.: Ueber Einklemmung bzw. Strangulation der Cauda equina, Deutsch. Med. Wschr. **35**:697, 1909.
[6]Dandy, W. E.: Loose cartilage from intervertebral disc simulating tumor of the spinal cord, Arch. Surg. **19**:660, 1929.
[7]Mixter, W. J., and Barr, J. S.: Rupture of the intervertebral disc with involvement of the spinal canal, New Eng. J. Med. **211**:210-215, 1934.

histories of 16 patients at the Massachusetts General Hospital with the diagnosis of enchondroma and found that the pathologic specimens in 10 of the persons consisted of intervertebral disc material. The role of the herniated disc in the etiology of sciatica was described by Mixter and Barr[7] in 1934. Over the next 10 years such neurosurgeons as Love, Spurling, Semmes, and Dandy reported their operative experiences with increasing numbers of patients. As early as 1938 Love and Walsh[8] had had experience with 100 surgical cases of disc disease. It was reported that well over half the patients were afforded complete relief of symptoms. By 1940 patients with severe sciatica who had not responded to conservative treatment were usually relieved by removal of the herniated discs. These early clinical reports of the short-term results of disc surgery seemed impressive, but the course beyond the immediate postconvalescent period remained unclear and the long-term history of intervertebral disc disease was vague even in patients treated conservatively.

HERNIATED LUMBAR DISC AND MILITARY SERVICE

Early military medical historians failed to mention backache or leg pain as an important disability among soldiers. Even World War I produced no reports concerning those disorders. Spurling[9] stated that "by the time the United States entered World War II, the clinical picture of the ruptured intervertebral disc was well established and diagnostic methods had become reasonably well standardized." Both conservative and surgical means to treat this disease were recognized, and hemilaminectomies, with removal of disc material, were common practice among neurosurgeons. Under medical surveillance in World War II were many men who either already harbored disc disease originating before entry into the Army or developed it after entry. The present report of a 20-year clinical follow-up is based on the Army experience with lumbar disc disease diagnosed during 1944-1945.

The method of treatment in the Army evolved through a series of policies beginning in the spring of 1942, when Spurling established the first neurosurgical service at Walter Reed General Hospital, Washington, D. C. Clinical policies for the treatment of disc disease were adopted for the United States and the overseas theaters. Mixter, acting for the Society of Neurological Surgeons, proposed to Fred W. Rankin, the Chief Surgical Consultant for the Office of the Surgeon General, that some Army and Navy hospitals be specified as centers for the diagnosis and treatment of disc disease. Neurosurgical services were to be set up for this purpose. A method of screening patients evolved in which a form on each patient with herniated nucleus pulposus (HNP) was submitted to the Neurosurgical Unit, and the patient was accepted or rejected for admission and clinical evaluation. The clinical evaluation of each patient was to include myelography, and the surgical treatment was to be standardized. Orthopedic surgeons and neurosurgeons had joint responsibility for selection of patients for surgery. The clinical manifestations were listed, and it was emphasized that "great discretion" was to be exercised in selecting patients for surgery. Two categories of patients were established, line-of-duty-yes (symptoms beginning in Army) and line-of-duty-no (symp-

[8]Love, J. G., and Walsh, M. N.: Protruded intervertebral discs: report of one hundred cases in which operation was performed, J.A.M.A. **111:**396-400, 1938.
[9]Spurling, R. G.: Management of the ruptured intervertebral disc (herniated nucleus pulposus). In United States Army, Surgery in World War II, vol. II, Neurosurgery, Washington, D. C., 1959, Office of the Surgeon General, Department of the Army.

toms beginning before induction). At this time the chief indication for surgery was intractable sciatic pain. With regard to preinduction disability, "no individual with a preinduction disability was to be considered for elective surgery unless he gave particular promise of being of future value to the Army from both the mental and the physical standpoint."[9]

In a statistical study the magnitude of the problem was examined on the basis of 483 enlisted personnel admitted to Army hospitals for HNP in 1943. The admission rate was about 0.5 per thousand strength. The analysis of treatment results in this group revealed that within 1 year of diagnosis 31% of the enlisted personnel treated surgically and 78% of those treated conservatively had been separated from service for medical reasons. During this time the surgical results in the Army were considered to be as favorable as those experienced in civilian practice. In the latter half of 1944 and during the first months of 1945, the situation changed and the late results of lumbar disc surgery, evaluated in relation to the return of personnel to active military duty, were recognized as unsatisfactory. It was then concluded: "There was no doubt, in short, that the results of surgery for ruptured disc in military practice were by no means as good as they were in civilian practice. The belief was also growing that practically all patients with ruptured discs, whether or not the disability existed before induction, were likely to have their symptoms aggravated by military service, and that line-of-duty evaluation should, therefore, play practically no part in the decision for or against operation."[9]

The Army policy in May 1944 specified that an enlisted man should be discharged if he was unable to "perform a reasonable day's work for the Army." Most men operated on for HNP were in that category. It was also proposed that the recent introduction of a stringent reconditioning system for rehabilitating men for return to duty was not suitable for patients with HNP. In March 1945 a reevaluation of results on 20% of the 1943 sample revealed a rise in the medical separation rate from 31% to 56% and an increase in the total separation rate postoperatively from 66% to 83%. Those figures were thought to represent the inability of patients with disc disease to withstand the rigors of Army life.

Finally, in 1945 the Army's policy was again changed as follows: "All patients with a diagnosis of HNP established as not in line-of-duty were to be treated conservatively and then separated from service in accordance for current military directive unless they desired surgery for intractable pain or there was evidence of neural paralysis. Military personnel who developed ruptures of the intervertebral disc in line-of-duty were to be treated with the objective of achieving maximum hospital benefit. Treatment was to be by conservative methods or, if the patient desired it, by surgery. After maximum hospital benefits had been attained, disposition was to be in accordance with current directives. The "inherent repetitive character" of the syndrome of herniated nucleus pulposus was to be closely examined in determining the line-of-duty status of each individual case."[9] Because of the end of the war there was little opportunity to put this policy into effect, but the changes reflect the basic lack of understanding of the life history of herniated disc disease.

IMPLEMENTATION OF THE CLINICAL STUDY OF LUMBAR HNP

The suggestion to study herniation of the nucleus pulposus was submitted to the Committee on Veterans Medical Problems of the National Research Council

(NRC) by the Office of the Surgeon General, U. S. Army, in a list of research topics for which veteran follow-up was particularly applicable.[10] Planning efforts were started in 1955. At the recommendation of Barnes Woodhall a follow-up examination program was established within the VA to be carried out on men hospitalized for lumbar disc lesions during World War II. The NRC Follow-up Agency (FUA) provided the mechanism for coordinating this effort.

A unit of the Division of Medical Sciences, the FUA provides a central focus for studies on the military-veteran population, enabling investigators to link the military and veteran periods in the interests of medical research. The program was started in 1946, following the recommendation of an NRC ad hoc Committee on Veterans Medical Problems.[10] In general the FUA collates information from military service records, the VA, other governmental agencies, private treatment facilities, and special questionnaires or medical examinations.[11]

Woodhall's experience in the Army and later in civilian practice convinced him that much remained to be learned about disc disease. Pointing to the lack of any systematic understanding of the natural history of HNP, and the limited nature of follow-up studies in civilian practice, he noted that a long-term VA study might have the following advantages:

1. The sampling situation was unique, in that one might hope for a virtually complete representation of men with symptomatic disc lesions of recent origin.
2. The World War II experience was large (about 14,000 cases with the diagnosis of HNP) with a follow-up period of at least 20 years.
3. The military experience created an exceptional opportunity for unbiased comparisons of men with and without symptomatic disc lesions.
4. The VA then compensated 16,000 World War II veterans for HNP incurred in or aggravated by military service, a number in excess of recorded World War II admissions.
5. Administrative considerations have governed treatment as much as or more than clinical considerations. This afforded some hope that unbiased treatment comparisons might be made on the basis of military material.
6. There was some expectation that a considerable fraction of any desired sample could be reexamined through the VA according to protocol, and that meaningful comparisons of volunteers and men who refused examination could be made by using existing documents available through the VA.

Woodhall also pointed out some disadvantages of such a long-term study:

1. The diagnosis was not easy or sure; thus a series attributable to a large number of individual medical officers would have to be reviewed from the standpoint of a single, uniform set of diagnostic criteria.
2. It seems generally supposed that the desire of some men to evade overseas service in time of war, or to return to civilian life, may have increased the usual difficulties of the diagnosis.

---

[10]Committee on Veterans Medical Problems, Division of Medical Sciences, National Academy of Sciences–National Research Council: Report on the value and feasibility of a long term program of follow-up study and clinical research, Washington, D. C., 28 June 1946.

[11]DeBakey, M. E., and Beebe, G. W.: Medical follow-up studies on veterans, J.A.M.A. **182:**1103-1109, 1962.

3. Evaluation of the significance of reported pain was made more difficult by the fact of service connection of and compensation for an appreciable proportion of cases.
4. Treatment comparisons on historical material were often difficult and usually unreliable; selection of cases for this purpose would have to rest on fixed, uniform criteria applied to the information on pretreatment status.

Later, in 1959, a protocol was developed by M. Dean Nefzger, of the FUA, and B. S. Nashold, Jr., which outlined the objectives of the study, gave procedures for selection of the sample and abstracting of information from medical records, and specified examination procedures. The subjects were to be examined by a group of neurosurgeons, neurologists, and orthopedic surgeons at seventeen VA hospitals. The clinical evaluations began in 1961 and lasted until 1964. During the later phases, the Social Work Service of the VA Central Office enlisted the help of social service staffs at local hospitals to interview patients who initially refused examination. At the conclusion of the clinical examinations a group of VA radiologists reviewed available radiographic materials.

CHAPTER *2*

MATERIALS AND METHODS

ZDENEK HRUBEC and BLAINE S. NASHOLD, JR.

SELECTION OF CLINICAL SAMPLE AND ABSTRACTING OF RECORDS

The sample used in this study was selected from punchcard files in the Office of the Surgeon General of the Army by identifying World War II hospital admissions for herniated nucleus pulposus. Altogether, 9,675 diagnoses of HNP were evaluated for eligibility. They were identified through 20% samples of hospital admissions during 1943-1946 and 100% of separations for HNP disability during 1943-1948. After the exclusion of those ineligible for the study on procedural or demographic criteria—164 females, 434 nonwhites, 6 with duplicate service numbers, 63 with incorrect service numbers or not found in file, 160 with first admissions after 1946, and 1,620 multiple HNP diagnoses for men otherwise eligible— there remained 7,228 men whose first service admission for HNP occurred during 1943-1946. On further evaluation the admission rosters for 1943 and 1946 were thought to be incomplete and were excluded. This left 4,872 cases with first admissions during 1944-1945, and they were used to select the sample for the clinical study.

Through a search of VA claims folders, 1,484 patients were identified whose most recent address was within traveling distance of one of the seventeen examining centers of the study. Their service and VA medical records were reviewed to further establish their eligibility and to abstract pertinent information. In this review 247 patients were excluded because their records did not support the selection criteria of this study—first service hospital admission for lumbar HNP during 1944-1945.* Another 114 patients, while otherwise eligible, resided in areas in which the capacity of the examining center was exceeded and therefore were not requested to participate in the examinations. The remaining 1,123 eligible patients compose the clinical sample. They were allocated for follow-up examination to the participating centers near which they resided. For this group, clinical information on service hospitalizations, data on demographic or socioeconomic variables, and results of the induction physical examination were abstracted from service records. Because of the possibility of multiple admissions during 1944-1945, the first Army admission for HNP is designated as the *reference hospitalization*. For 54% of the patients it was also possible to obtain the Army roentgenograms from the reference hospitalization pertaining to the back. The records of the reference hospitalization indicated that 93% of the patients had had roentgenograms of the spine. The availability of the films for our study was determined by the extent to which the Army

---

*The reasons for exclusion and the number of patients found ineligible due to each are: diagnosed as having HNP before 1944 (103), final hospital diagnosis was not HNP of the lumbar spine (70), evidence of surgery for HNP before entering service (10), and for other miscellaneous reasons (64).

pursued specific film disposal procedures. These probably did not introduce much bias with respect to important clinical variables. For example, films were available for 57% of patients with surgery for HNP at the reference hospitalization and for 53% of patients without such surgery.

ACQUISITION OF FOLLOW-UP DATA

Contacting patients and asking them to be examined was the responsibility of the clinical participants at each examination center. As a part of the allocation procedure, the clinical participants were provided with copies of the pertinent portions of all hospital records, the original Army roentgenograms, and appropriate forms and instructions for recording the results of the follow-up examination. Samples of these materials are included in the Appendix (pp. 71 to 97).

The examination consisted of family and personal medical history, specific questions about symptoms of disc disease, careful evaluation of neurologic and mechanical signs of HNP, and an overall evaluation of the patient's disability. Roentgenograms of the lumbar spine were prepared by the radiology departments of the participating VA hospitals. As a part of the history obtained at follow-up, patients were asked about private hospital admissions since service. The VA claims folders contained information on any VA hospitalizations, and for patients receiving compensation, on all other hospitalizations as well. When private hospitalizations were reported, an attempt was made to obtain copies of the pertinent hospital records. To avoid variation in the likelihood of detecting a follow-up hospitalization as a result of different dates of examination, 30 June 1961, when the examination program was started, was chosen as the *cutoff date* for considering follow-up data on hospitalizations.

At the conclusion of the clinical phase of the study, the Army and VA roentgenograms of the lumbar spine were reviewed by a group of eight radiologists, who evaluated 418 Army films and 760 films obtained at the follow-up examination. Army films were included in the review only if follow-up films were available. In addition to those film reviews, each reviewer independently evaluated several films processed as a part of the routine review by another radiologist. The reviewers could not distinguish the films processed twice from those processed only once. The duplicate reviews provided a basis for a methodologic evaluation of the reliability of the radiographic review.

RELEVANT CHARACTERISTICS OF STUDY SUBJECTS

In the sample of 1,123 patients who were allocated for examination, 92% had filed claims for disability with the VA and 79% were receiving compensation on 30 June 1961. The median year of birth of these patients was 1915. The median age at reference hospital admission was 29.8 years, which is considerably greater than the median ages of men in the Army in 1944 and 1945—24.1 and 20.2 years, respectively. Among the study cases, 9.2% were commissioned officers. In the total Army in 1944, commissioned officers constituted 9.7%.

Of the 1,123 patients in this sample, 395 experienced some kind of surgical intervention for HNP at the reference hospitalization.* The distribution of patients

---

*Five other operations were performed at the reference hospitalization but cannot be considered as operations for HNP, since they were described as exploratory, rhizotomy, decompression of nerve root, etc.

Table 2-1. Percent age distribution by surgical status in study sample, Army admissions for herniated nucleus pulposus, 1944-1945

Age at reference hospitalization	No surgery	Surgery for HNP	Other surgery	Total
0–19	1.5	2.5	–	1.9
20–24	17.0	21.3	–	18.4
25–29	29.9	32.7	–	31.0
30–34	28.9	25.3	–	27.6
35–39	19.2	15.9	–	18.1
40+	3.5	2.3	–	3.0
Total	100.0	100.0	–	100.0
Number	723	395	5	1,123
Median age (yr.)	30.3	29.0	–	29.8

Table 2-2. Number of patients in study sample by VA examining center and disposition

VA examining center	Allocated	Examined	Refused examination	Not located, other	Percent examined
Albany	28	21	6	1	75.0
Boston	90	67	20	3	74.4
Bronx	113	81	24	8	71.7
Chicago	106	59	36	11	55.7
Coral Gables	42	32	9	1	76.2
Denver	26	22	3	1	84.6
Durham	56	45	9	2	80.4
Hines	47	35	12	0	74.5
Long Beach	127	77	24	26	60.6
Minneapolis	55	48	7	0	87.3
New Orleans	20	20	0	0	100.0
New York	78	29	35	14	37.2
Philadelphia	73	49	17	7	67.1
Pittsburgh	85	59	25	1	69.4
Richmond	37	32	2	3	86.5
San Francisco	100	82	8	10	82.0
Seattle	40	31	6	3	77.5
Total	1,123	789	243	91	70.3

Table 2-3. Percent and number of patients in study sample by relevant admissions after reference hospitalization and examination status

Relevant follow-up hospitalization*	Examined at follow-up	Refused examination	Not located or other not examined	Total	Number
None	63.2	27.9	8.9	100.0	584
Service, after reference hospital	71.8	10.7	17.5	100.0	103
VA or VA contract, no service	80.1	17.1	2.8	100.0	251
Private only	82.9	12.2	4.9	100.0	41
Hospitalization not relevant or unknown status	77.1	14.6	8.3	100.0	144
Total	70.3	21.6	8.1	100.0	1,123

*Before the cutoff date, 30 June 1961, related to disc disease.

by operation status and age at the reference hospitalization is shown in Table 2-1. Among the 728 not operated on for HNP at the reference hospitalization, 13.9% were operated on for HNP during the follow-up period. In the total sample, 14.2% were operated on for HNP during this time. There were 539 patients who had further hospital admissions during the follow-up period before the cutoff date of 30 June 1961. However, for 144 of these, the relevance of the hospital admission to lumbar disc disease could not be established. Of the 979 patients with known status, 40.3% were admitted for disc disease during the follow-up period.

In the entire sample, 1,032 patients could be located at the address available to us. Of that number, 789 (76.5%) were examined and 40 of those refusing participation were interviewed by social service workers. In the total sample of 1,123 eligible subjects, the examination rate was 70.3%. The percentage of patients examined at follow-up is shown by hospital in Table 2-2. The examination rate varied somewhat among examining centers and tended to be lower in the large cities. The rate also varied with different characteristics of the patients. Among those receiving VA disability compensation it was 74.3% compared to 47.6% among those without such compensation. Of men born in the years 1905 to 1909, 75.8% were examined at follow-up, whereas in the one older and four younger age groups, the examination rate did not exceed 70.0%. Among commissioned officers 51.5% were examined, whereas among enlisted men the rate was 72.2%. Differences in examination rates with age are not statistically significant, but those with VA disability compensation and rank are significant (P <.001 and P <.01, respectively).

A distribution of patients by type of follow-up hospitalization and by examination status is given in Table 2-3. Among men not hospitalized in the follow-up period 63.2% were examined, whereas among men who were hospitalized for back or leg complaints the rate of follow-up examination is 78.2% (P <.001). The rate of follow-up examinations for the 395 patients with HNP surgery at the reference hospitalization is 78.7%. Among the remaining 728 patients 65.7% were examined (P <.001). In Chapter 6, Table 6-1, the clinical findings during the reference hospitalization are compared for those with and those without a follow-up examination.

SUMMARY

With the use of punchcard files of Army hospital admissions in World War II, 1,123 men were identified who resided within convenient traveling distance from one of the examination centers of the study, whose first service admission for lumbar HNP was during 1944-1945, and who met the other selective criteria. The first hospitalization in the 1944-1945 period has been designated as the *reference hospitalization*. The service medical records of this hospitalization have been reviewed and abstracted along with other service and VA records, and for more than half the patients reference hospital roentgenograms of the lumbar spine were recovered. Of the 1,123 patients, 789 were examined between 1961 and 1964 according to a standard protocol, and roentgenograms of the lumbar spine were obtained at that time. The rates of examination vary somewhat with examining center, surgical status, and other characteristics of the subjects. The examined patients are more likely to be compensated for disability, to have had surgery at the reference hospitalization, to have served as enlisted men, and to reside in or around the smaller cities compared to those who could not be examined.

CHAPTER 3

CLINICAL HISTORY AND SYMPTOMS

BLAINE S. NASHOLD, JR., and ZDENEK HRUBEC

FAMILY HISTORY

At the follow-up examination, 789 men were evaluated clinically, and an additional 40 men were interviewed by social service workers but were not examined. Specific replies regarding family history were obtained for 808 of the 829. A positive family history of low back pain was reported by 21.5% of the respondents. Sciatica and operations for lumbar HNP were noted less often than was a history of low back pain. There was a higher frequency of positive reports of low back pain for fathers than for mothers, and a higher frequency for brothers than for sisters. A predominance of impairments of the back and spine and of lumbar disc disease in males has been noted before, but a family relationship has not been noted in previous studies of disc disease and is neither suggested nor contradicted by these data.[1-3]

The personal medical histories of the patients were obtained during the follow-up examination to evaluate possible clues for other connective tissue disease. The following percentages of patients reported specific diseases of interest: bursitis, 18.3%; hypertrophic arthritis, 15.2%; urinary calculi, 8.6%; cervical disc rupture, 4.4%; thoracic disc rupture, 1.0%; compression of ulnar or median nerves, 2.8%; hip disease, 3.3%; periarticular fibrosis and shoulder-arm syndrome, 1.5%. The histories of cervical and thoracic disc rupture were often supported by diagnostic information in the available medical records. The unexpectedly high frequencies do not result from mistakes in reporting the level of herniation and suggest a more fundamental relationship with lumbar disc disease. However, the other conditions are relatively common and the percentages reported may be comparable to those in the population free of disc disease.

ONSET OF BACK AND LEG PAIN

The hospital records of all cases except one indicated either back pain or leg pain at the time of the reference hospitalization. Of the 1,123 men in the sample, only 27 were free of back pain and 24 were free of leg pain. The remaining 1,073 patients, or 95.5%, experienced pain in both back and legs at the onset of the

---

[1]Spurling, R. G., and Grantham, E. G.: The end-results of surgery for ruptured intervertebral discs; follow-up study of 327 cases, J. Neurosurg. **6**:57-64, 1949.

[2]Barr, J. S.: Ruptured intervertebral disc and sciatic pain, J. Bone Joint Surg. **29**:429-437, 1947.

[3]U. S. Department of Health, Education, and Welfare, National Center for Health Statistics: Chronic conditions causing activity limitation, United States—July 1963-June 1965, PHS Pub. no. 1000, series 10, no. 51, Washington, D. C., Feb. 1969, U. S. Government Printing Office.

illness that led to the reference hospitalization. The left leg was the site of the *first attack* of pain more frequently (45.0%) than the right (36.1%). At the onset of the episode leading to the reference hospital admission, leg pain was present on the left in 48.4% of the patients and on the right in 39.5%. This tendency to more frequent involvement of the left side has been confirmed by other investigators.[4] The duration of pain varied considerably. A few patients had their first attack of pain during the reference hospitalization. The year of onset of back pain could not be determined for 34 patients, and the year of onset of leg pain could not be determined for 62, either because there was no pain at that site or because the year of onset had not been recorded.

The distribution of the year of onset of pain in the back and legs is given in Table 3-1. Leg pain appeared more often than back pain in the 1944-1945 period in which the hospitalizations occurred. Only 11.7% of the patients had onset of leg pain 5 or more years before 1944-1945, but the proportion with back pain of this duration is 28.6%. Table 3-2 indicates the nature of onset of disc symptoms as beginning with either back or leg pain by the duration of back pain prior to admission. At the time of admission only 9.8% had back pain, and 25.6% had leg pain of less than 2 months' duration.* For most patients back pain preceded leg pain. Only 39 patients had onset of leg pain before back pain. For 56 patients the sequence of onset of pain could not be determined. For the others, Table 3-2 indicates that, as one would expect, when back pain occurred before leg pain a high proportion of patients had back pain of long duration. In fact, when symptoms started with leg pain the onset was likely to be considerably more recent than when back pain occurred first. Among the 39 patients whose first symptom was leg pain, 64.1% had the disease for less than 2 years and 46.2% for less than 1 year. Among the 603 patients whose first symptom was back pain 44.8% had the disease for less than 2 years and 29.5% for less than 1 year. The differences are statistically significant (P <.05). In the group with simultaneous onset of back and leg pain the disease appeared to be of intermediate duration. Among all men for whom the duration of leg pain was known (1,061), onset of leg pain occurred within 3 months of the reference hospital admission in 33.9%. It seems reasonable that the appearance of leg pain frequently precipitated hospitalization and diagnosis of HNP.

Bilateral leg pain occurred more often with longer duration of symptoms. Among patients with onset of *back pain* in 1942 or earlier, 13.3% had leg pain in both legs at the reference hospitalization (usually simultaneously but sometimes alternately), whereas among men with a more recent onset of back pain only 6.6% had bilateral leg symptoms (P <.001). Similarly, among patients whose *leg pain* first occurred in 1942 or earlier, bilateral leg symptoms were manifested at the reference hospitalization in 14.1%; among men with a more recent onset of leg pain, it was bilateral in only 8.7% (P <.02). In Table 3-2 it was shown that the onset of back pain represented the onset of symptoms for a large majority of patients. Since the

---

[4]Hanraets, P. R. M. J.: The degenerative back and its differential diagnosis, Amsterdam, 1959, Elsevier Publishing Co.

*The interval from onset of back pain to reference hospitalization as determined from the history at that admission had a mean value of 46.1 months, a median value of 23.2 months, and a range of zero to 294 months. The interval from onset of leg pain had a mean value of 22.4 months, a median of 5.4 months, and a range of zero to 369 months.

Table 3-1. Percent and number by year of first attack of pain and by site determined from history at the reference hospitalization in 1944-1945

Year of onset	Back		Leg	
	Percent	Number	Percent	Number
<1930	3.4	38	1.0	11
1930–1934	6.9	78	2.3	26
1935–1939	18.3	206	8.4	94
1940–1942	18.7	210	11.7	131
1943	15.5	174	15.2	171
1944	21.6	243	33.4	375
1945	12.5	140	22.5	253
None or unknown	3.0	34	5.5	62
Total	99.9	1,123	100.0	1,123

Table 3-2. Percent of patients by interval from first attack of back pain to the reference hospitalization and sequence of onset of back and leg pain

Interval: onset of back pain to reference hospitalization	Sequence of symptom onset				Total
	Leg before back	Leg and back simultaneously	Back before leg	Other or unknown	
0–5 months	53.8	29.9	17.2	23.1	23.5
6–11 months	28.2	11.0	12.3	2.6	12.0
1 year and over	18.0	59.1	70.5	74.3	64.5
Total	100.0	100.0	100.0	100.0	100.0
Number—interval known	39	408	603	39	1,089
Unknown interval or no back pain	0	1	16	17	34

reference hospital admissions took place in 1944-1945, patients with onset of back pain in 1942 or earlier can be considered chronic.

Various activities such as lifting, bending, jumping, calisthenics, coughing, falling, etc., were mentioned as being associated with the onset of the first episode of pain in the back or in the legs. Some activity was mentioned in the records as being associated with 76% of the onsets of back pain and 62% of the onsets of leg pain. Of all the records, 9% stated explicitly that no activities were associated with the onset of back pain, and in 15%, activity at onset was not mentioned. Explicit statements of no activity at onset of leg pain were made in 11% of the records, and 27% did not mention activity at onset. With respect to the onset of either leg or back pain, the two most frequently mentioned factors were lifting (loading) and falls (jumps). The frequency with which these activities at onset were reported did not vary appreciably with year of onset of back pain, leg pain, or sequence of onset of leg and back pain.

CLINICAL FINDINGS AND COURSE AT THE REFERENCE HOSPITAL

Among cases operated on during the reference hospitalization there was a tendency toward short intervals between onset of leg pain and the hospital admission. Of patients operated on for HNP during the reference hospitalization, 55.4% had onset of leg pain less than 6 months before admission, whereas of those

Table 3-3. Percent of patients by interval from onset of back pain to the reference hospitalization and by operation status

Interval: onset of back pain to reference hospitalization	Operation status		Total	Number
	No HNP operation at reference hospital	HNP operation at reference hospital		
0–5 months	56.6	43.4	100.0	256
6–11 months	58.0	42.0	100.0	131
1 year	64.3	35.7	100.0	154
2 + years	70.4	29.6	100.0	548
Unknown or no back pain	64.7	35.3	100.0	34
Total	64.8	35.2	100.0	1,123

Table 3-4. Percent of patients by restriction of spine motion during the reference hospitalization and by side of pain in legs

Limitation of back motion	Side of pain in legs			Total	Number of patients
	Right	Left	Neither or both		
Right bending	60.4	29.2	10.3	99.9	106
Left bending	23.2	71.2	5.6	100.0	125

not operated on, 44.3% were in this category (P <.001). Long intervals were found more often among patients with no operations during the reference hospitalization. An evaluation of operation status in relation to back pain is summarized in Table 3-3. Among those with onset of back pain within 6 months of admission, proportionately more patients were operated on for HNP during the reference hospitalization than among those with earlier onset (P <.001); this relationship is comparable to the one noted for duration of leg pain.

Those whose back pain and leg pain occurred simultaneously were operated on for HNP during the reference hospitalization less frequently (27.1%) than those whose back pain occurred before the leg pain (40.4%, P <.001). Those with simultaneous onset had a somewhat higher frequency of first operations for HNP in the follow-up period (11.7%) than the other onset groups (7.5%, P <.05).

The results of sciatic palpation to determine tenderness were not uniformly recorded during the reference hospitalization. There was no mention of the procedure in 48% of the service medical records. Among the patients for whom the item was complete, the left leg was involved slightly more frequently (45.1%) than the right (35.9%). The results of localized percussion of the back were not recorded in 57% of the records. When the latter records are excluded, there is a positive association between operations for HNP during the reference hospitalization and the proportion of positive localized percussion findings. In the group operated on, 66.2% had positive findings; in those never operated on, 57.3% had positive findings.

Of the 1,030 patients whose records specified the extent of spine motion, 97.6% exhibited some restriction. Lateral motion was restricted only to the right or only to the left for 231 patients. Table 3-4 shows the strong positive association between the side of leg pain and side of restriction of spine motion.

Information on spine contour was obtained during the reference hospitalization for 702 of the 1,123 patients. There was no appreciable difference in the frequency with which scoliosis was found by year of onset of back pain. The sequence of pain onset in legs or back in the total group appeared unrelated to presence of scoliosis, but within the group with recent onset, 1943-1945, those whose back pain preceded leg pain had a somewhat higher percentage of scoliosis (53.7%) than those whose back and leg pain occurred simultaneously (42.5%).

The extent of leg pain during attacks before the reference hospitalization has been specified for 996 patients. No striking associations were evident between the extent of leg pain and the sequence of pain onset or operation status. However, those with recent onset of back pain, during the years 1943-1945, included a slightly but significantly (P <.01) lower fraction with leg pain extending only to the knee (11.5%) than those whose back pain started before 1943 (17.8%). There was only a slight association between the level of lesion diagnosed at the reference hospital admission and the extent of pain. The proportion of patients with foot and toe pain was 54.1% when the diagnosis specified the L5-S1 level and 47.9% when it specified the L4-L5 level. The difference is not significant.

There was a strong association between the side of leg pain and the side of the HNP diagnosis. For 71.2% of the 972 patients for whom both level of diagnosis and side of leg pain were known, there was exact agreement between the statement of the laterality of pain (right leg, left leg, bilateral) with the laterality of the diagnosis. If the definition of agreement is extended so that the bilateral designation on one classification is considered to agree with either the right, left, or bilateral designations on the other classification, this figure increases to 98.1%.

PAIN IN RELATION TO OTHER CLINICAL FINDINGS AT THE FOLLOW-UP EXAMINATION

Follow-up examinations were done in 789 patients, and status with respect to back pain or sciatica was determined for 782. Another 40 patients were evaluated by social service interviews. Of the patients whose status was evaluated, 85.9% reported some degree of back pain at the follow-up examination, 61.2% reported some degree of leg pain, and 6.8% were altogether free of pain. However, only 14.6% of the patients characterized the back pain as severe and only 9.6% reported severe sciatica. The percentage of patients with sciatic pain is shown by presence and severity of back pain in Table 3-5. The same degree of severity tends to be reported by the patient for both back pain and sciatica. Patients operated on for HNP during the reference hospitalization had a somewhat lower frequency of simultaneous back pain and sciatica at follow-up (47.7%) than did nonsurgical patients (58.0%, P <.005). The frequency of back pain did not differ appreciably with surgical status, and the above difference is due primarily to the relationship of sciatica with surgical status shown in Table 3-6.

Status with respect to motor, sensory, and reflex signs was determined at the follow-up examination for 743 patients. The completeness with which this information was obtained did not vary excessively with year of onset of back pain or with the presence or absence of bilateral leg pain at the reference hospitalization. Among patients with onset of back pain before 1942, 37.0% exhibited simultaneously motor, sensory, and reflex signs at follow-up; among those with back pain of shorter duration, 30.2% exhibited this combination of signs. The difference is not large and is of marginal significance (P <.06). When all sign status groups

Table 3-5. Percent of patients with sciatic pain by presence and severity of back pain determined at the follow-up examination

Sciatic pain at follow-up	Back pain at follow-up				
	None	Mild	Moderate	Severe	Total
None	48.3*	46.2	34.6	20.0	38.8
Mild	24.1	43.9	21.7	21.7	30.5
Moderate	15.5	6.7	39.3	22.5	21.0
Severe	12.1	3.2	4.4	35.8	9.6
Total percent	100.0	100.0	100.0	100.0	99.9
Number	116	314	272	120	822

*Categories indicating same degree of back and sciatic pain are italicized.

Table 3-6. Percent distribution of sciatica at the follow-up examination by surgical status at the reference hospitalization

Sciatic pain	Surgery for HNP	No surgery for HNP	Total
None	44.7	34.9	38.8
Mild	28.6	31.8	30.5
Moderate	18.8	22.5	21.0
Severe	7.9	10.8	9.6
Total	100.0	100.0	99.9
Number with known status	329	493	822
Number with unknown status	66	235	301

are considered, the two distributions by year of onset of back pain are similar. The distribution of signs at the follow-up examination was also evaluated by side of leg pain at the reference hospitalization, and no remarkable differences were found among those with right, left, or bilateral pain. Likewise, no differences in the motor, sensory, and reflex findings were found with the sequence of onset of back pain and leg pain.

SUMMARY

This study is the first to point out a predominance of positive family histories of low back pain in male relatives compared with female relatives. However, this finding is consistent with the previously reported higher prevalence among males. Sciatica or operations for lumbar HNP were noted less often among family members than was a positive history of low back pain. In the patient's own medical history, reports of cervical and thoracic disc disease were unusually frequent, and it was often possible to verify the history in the available medical records. Also of interest was the occurrence of other diseases of connective tissue origin, such as bursitis, hypertrophic arthritis, ulnar and median nerve compression, hip disease, periarticular fibrosis, and shoulder-arm syndrome.

The initial symptom of lumbar HNP seems to be pain. Generally occurring first in the back and then in the leg, pain was reported by all but one patient at the reference hospital admission, and 95.5% had pain in both back and legs. The physical activities most often associated with the first attack were lifting, loading, jumping, or falling. Leg pain occurred more commonly on the left than on the right. If the first attack started with leg pain, it was likely to have been more recent than if it started with back pain. We believe that the patients were hospitalized for HNP primarily because of leg pain. There was a tendency for it to occur in both legs, particularly if leg pain was of a long duration. There was a slight tendency for foot and toe pain to be associated with a disc lesion at the L5-S1 level rather than at the L4-L5 level, but the relationship was not sufficiently consistent to provide a means of diagnosing the level.

The clinical findings during the reference hospitalization verified the anamnestic history. Pain associated with sciatic nerve tenderness to palpation occurred more frequently on the left than on the right; and on percussion when the results were recorded, spinal lumbar pain was a common finding. Spinal motion was restricted in almost all patients, who were more often unable to tilt their spine toward the painful leg without aggravating it than to tilt it in the opposite direction.

The clinical findings after 20 years reveal that some degree of either back or leg pain persists in most patients. However, severe sciatica or back pain is not common. Patients who were operated on for HNP during the reference hospitalization experienced leg pain at follow-up somewhat less often than the nonsurgical patients. At the follow-up examination, no differences in the motor, sensory, and reflex changes were found in relation to the sequence of onset of the initial back or leg pain.

CHAPTER 4

CLINICAL SIGNS BY PHYSICAL EXAMINATION

CHARLES B. WILSON

This chapter evaluates observations obtained at the time of the reference hospitalization before the *reference date*. The latter is defined as the date of surgery if this occurs within 90 days of admission. For nonsurgical patients and for those with later surgery, it is the day 3 months after admission for HNP. Also evaluated here are observations obtained at the follow-up examination 20 years later according to a standard protocol. The observations are conveniently categorized as postural and neurologic signs. Postural signs are related to the mechanics of spinal posture and movement and to the condition of the lumbar paravertebral muscles. Neurologic signs include motor, sensory, and reflex abnormalities in the legs. The results of two tests—straight leg raising and jugular compression—are included under neurologic signs. For definition of terms and methods of examination, see Appendix (pp. 80 to 95).

The frequency of different signs is examined in this chapter in relation to the occurrence of others determined at the same period of observation—during the reference hospitalization and at the follow-up examination. The frequency of each sign is also evaluated in relation to the surgical status of the patient during the reference hospitalization and during the follow-up period. In addition, analyses of special relevance to specific signs are presented. No attempt is made here to predict the occurrence of signs at follow-up from the data of the reference hospitalization. The significance of the differences has been evaluated by the conventional chi-square test, and for each sign the results of certain of these tests are summarized in a tabular presentation. In the latter comparisons the corresponding probability levels have been omitted from the text.

POSTURAL SIGNS
Scoliosis and spinal tilt

During the reference hospitalization, scoliosis and spinal tilt had the following frequencies of occurrence: scoliosis alone, 20.7%; spinal tilt alone, 34.6%; scoliosis and spinal tilt, 32.1%; neither, 12.7%. The right-hand column of Table 4-1 indicates that the ascertainment of these signs at the reference hospitalization is more complete among the more disabled patients. More so than scoliosis, spinal tilt was strongly related to the other spinal abnormalities. The comparisons presented in Table 4-1 have been evaluated for significance and the results are summarized in Table 4-6. The frequency of scoliosis as diagnosed radiographically (27.0%) was lower than that observed on clinical examination (52.8%). Spinal tilt was more prevalent among patients who had been operated on during the reference hospitalization for HNP (72.4%) than among those who had not been operated on (63.5%) as indicated in Table 4-7.

Table 4-1. Percent with lumbar scoliosis, with spinal tilt, and with unknown status by status on other postural signs. Findings during reference hospitalization before reference date

Status on other signs	Percent with scoliosis	Percent with list or tilt	Number with known* status	Percent with unknown* status
Paravertebral muscle spasm	54.5	68.5	543	27.8
No paravertebral muscle spasm	47.6	58.8	143	52.2
Unknown status	43.8	75.0	16	77.8
Loss of lordosis	54.8	70.6	449	25.9
No loss of lordosis	49.8	58.7	237	46.7
Unknown status	43.8	75.0	16	77.8
Restricted flexion, extension, and lateral bending or rotation	53.4	78.4	264	22.8
Stated as restricted in all directions	57.3	61.9	131	33.5
Other multiple restriction	55.7	59.6	176	42.3
Flexion only restricted	36.8	58.5	106	43.0
Unknown status	60.0	48.0	25	73.1
Total	52.8	66.7	702	37.5

*Status during reference hospitalization with respect to the scoliosis–list-tilt classification was known for 702 and unknown for 421 men. Percent with unknown status = 100 • (1123-702)/1123 = 37.5, for example.

Scoliosis with convexity of the lumbar spine to the left was recorded for 152 patients and to the right for 108 (P <.01). There was only a slight opposite tendency to one-sidedness of spinal tilt, 190 to the left and 206 to the right; but, unlike scoliosis, tilt was strongly associated with leg pain on the opposite side. Of 359 patients for whom leg pain and side of tilt were specified as either to the right only or to the left only, 60.2% had leg pain on the opposite side and 39.8% had leg pain on the same side (P <.001). When there was pain in both legs, the percentage of patients with tilt was somewhat lower (58.0%) than when a single leg was involved (67.9%); this difference is not significant. These findings suggest that the mechanisms responsible for spinal tilt or scoliosis are not directly related to the side of the herniated disc but appear to be due to other undetermined manifestations of disc disease.

At the follow-up examination, scoliosis was noted more often when the patient was erect (14.0%) than when he was prone (5.7%). These observations were strongly associated with paravertebral muscle spasm, loss of lumbar lordosis, and restricted spinal motion, as indicated in Table 4-2 and 4-6. Patients with simultaneous restriction of flexion, extension, and lateral bending or spinal rotation had a much higher frequency of scoliosis (26.5%) than patients with no restriction of spinal motion (4.0%). There was no association between the operative status during the reference hospitalization or the follow-up period and scoliosis at the follow-up examination. The frequency of list or tilt at the follow-up examination was only 1.8%, which is not sufficient for a detailed evaluation of this sign. The results of statistical tests on scoliosis and tilt are presented in Tables 4-6 and 4-7.

Table 4-2. Percent with lumbar scoliosis of the spine by status on other postural signs. Findings at follow-up examination

Status on other signs	Percent with scoliosis	Number with known status	Number with unknown status*
Paravertebral muscle spasm	29.0	93	0
No paravertebral muscle spasm	11.7	685	3
Unknown status	—	5	3
Loss of lordosis	19.8	237	0
No loss of lordosis	11.1	541	3
Unknown status	—	5	3
Restriction of flexion, extension, and lateral bending or rotation	26.5	181	2
Flexion and lateral bending or rotation	14.1	99	2
Extension and lateral bending or rotation	12.5	120	0
Only lateral bending, rotation, or both	10.3	156	1
Only flexion, extension, or both	9.2	87	0
No restriction	4.0	100	0
Unknown status	12.5	40	1
Total	14.0	783	6

*Among 789 patients examined at follow-up.

The close correlation between the finding of spinal tilt and restricted spinal motion at the reference hospitalization agrees with general experience. Two thirds (66.7%) of all patients had a spinal tilt, but in only one third (32.1%) was an associated scoliosis noted. We doubt the existence of spinal tilt without some degree of compensatory scoliosis and consequently would consider this group of "spinal tilt" patients as having minimal rather than no scoliosis.

Scoliosis without spinal tilt was observed initially in 20.7% of patients. The poor correlation between scoliosis and other abnormal findings suggests that scoliosis without observable spinal tilt represents a mild postural manifestation of lumbar disc disease. The disappearance of scoliosis in the prone position seen at the follow-up examination reflects its dynamic nature as a postural compensating mechanism, rather than a structural change in the spine. A separation of spinal tilt and scoliosis in terms of their significance in disc disease finds some support in these data. Spinal tilt, with or without scoliosis, constitutes strong evidence of postural alteration, whereas scoliosis without spinal tilt does not. The high frequency of postural spinal deformity in disc disease (87.3%) confirms earlier reports.[1]

Paravertebral muscle spasm

Paravertebral muscle spasm was present in 71.6% of men during the reference hospitalization and was most frequently noted in patients with other mechanical signs. It was found in 78.9% of those having loss of lumbar lordosis compared to its occurrence in 61.6% of patients with normal lordosis. It was found in 82.6%

---

[1]Hanraets, P. R. M. J.: The degenerative back and its differential diagnosis, Amsterdam, 1959, Elsevier Publishing Co.

of those whose spine flexion, extension, and lateral bending or rotation were all restricted compared with 62.1% among those whose only restriction was on forward flexion. A slightly higher frequency of paravertebral muscle spasm occurred among patients selected for HNP operation (76.5%) during the reference hospitalization than among those who did not undergo such surgery (68.8%). The results of statistical testing of these comparisons are given in Tables 4-6 and 4-7.

At the follow-up examination, paravertebral muscle spasm was observed in 11.9%. It was found more frequently in patients with decreased lumbar lordosis (19.8%) and restricted rotation or lateral bending (14.8%) than among those free of these signs (8.5% and 3.2%, respectively). Paravertebral muscle spasm was found in 18.7% of the patients who exhibited simultaneously motor, sensory, and reflex signs, but in only 4.1% of those free of any of these signs (P <.001). The increase in the frequency of muscle spasm was about equal for the different kinds of neurologic involvement of the legs. The percentage of muscle spasm at the follow-up examination was unaffected by the operative status at the reference hospitalization or during the follow-up period (Table 4-7).

Although paravertebral muscle spasm occurs in a variety of traumatic and nontraumatic disorders of the spine, it is generally present in individuals with lumbar disc disease. During the reference hospitalization, paravertebral muscle spasm occurred quite frequently (71.6%), and at the follow-up examination, in the symptomatic patients, it was not an uncommon finding. Thus it seems to reflect some abnormality of the lumbar spine. Furthermore, the relative absence of muscle spasm in asymptomatic patients known to have abnormal lumbar discs indicates the reliability of paravertebral muscle spasm as an indication of symptomatic disc disease. Paravertebral muscle spasm appears to be a significant physical finding.

Loss of lumbar lordosis

A loss of lumbar lordosis was recorded for 57.7% during the reference hospitalization. Loss of lordosis was more frequent (72.3%) in patients with restricted flexion, extension, and rotation or lateral bending than in patients with less extensive restrictions (52.7%). The significance of this difference and of the relationships with other mechanical signs and with surgical status is summarized in Tables 4-6 and 4-7. Loss of lumbar lordosis was more frequent among patients operated on either during the reference hospitalization (65.9%) or during the follow-up period (64.4%) than among those not operated on for HNP during the reference hospitalization (52.6%). It was somewhat more frequent (69.3%) in patients with abnormal motor, sensory, and reflex signs than in patients who lacked some or all of these signs (56.0%, P <.005).

At follow-up, loss of lumbar lordosis was seen in 30.3% of the examined patients. Restricted spinal motion and a loss of lordosis were strongly associated; the greater the limitation of spinal motion, the higher the rate of loss of lordosis. Only 11.0% of the patients with no restrictions of spinal motion showed loss of lordosis. Patients operated on in the follow-up period had a higher frequency of loss of lordosis at follow-up (41.7%) than nonsurgical patients (27.4%). There was no significant difference in the frequency of loss of lordosis at follow-up with operative experience during the reference hospitalization (Table 4-7).

In the evaluation of lumbar disc disease, loss of lumbar lordosis has limited importance, although it was observed more frequently among patients with spinal list or tilt, paravertebral muscle spasm, or restricted spinal motion and among those with abnormal neurologic signs. There is some variation in the lumbar disc curve among patients without lumbar disc disease; and, although 57.7% of the patients exhibited loss of lumbar lordosis during the reference hospitalization, its presence does not strongly confirm the diagnosis of lumbar disc disease.

Restriction of lumbar spinal motion

Spinal motion has been categorized as not restricted; restricted on forward flexion; backward extension; rotation to right and left, or lateral flexion to right and left, or combinations thereof; or as stated to be limited in all directions. During the reference hospitalization, a variety of combinations of restriction occurred. Of 102 patients with limitation of rotation to either right or left, 81 also had restricted lateral flexion. When there was restriction of flexion or rotation to the

Table 4-3. Percent distribution of combinations of restriction of spinal motion. Findings during reference hospitalization before reference date

Restriction of spinal motion	Number	Percent
None	25	2.2
Flexion only	186	16.6
Extension only	17	1.5
Lateral bending and/or rotation only	9	0.8
Flexion and extension	103	9.2
Flexion and lateral bending and/or rotation	112	10.0
Extension and lateral bending and/or rotation	39	3.5
Flexion, extension, and lateral bending and/or rotation	342	30.4
Stated as limited in all directions	197	17.5
Unknown status	93	8.3
Total	1,123	100.0

Table 4-4. Percent distribution of restriction of spinal motion by status on other postural signs. Findings during reference hospitalization before reference date

Other sign status	Flexion, extension, and lateral bending or rotation*	Flexion and extension	Flexion only limited	Other restriction	No restriction	Total	Number with known status	Number with unknown status
Paravertebral muscle spasm	58.8	9.5	14.7	16.1	0.8	99.9	712	40
No paravertebral muscle spasm	40.6	11.3	23.2	19.5	5.4	100.0	276	23
Loss of lordosis	60.0	9.7	13.5	16.0	0.8	100.0	587	19
No loss of lordosis	44.4	10.5	22.4	18.7	4.0	100.0	401	44
No spasm and no loss of lordosis	35.1	11.3	22.5	23.2	7.9	100.0	151	20
Unknown status	21.4	9.5	40.5	19.1	9.5	100.0	42	30
Total	52.3	10.0	18.1	17.2	2.4	100.0	1,030	93

*Includes statement that restriction was in all directions.

Table 4-5. Percent distribution of lateral spinal motion observed before reference date by side of diagnosis of disc lesion and source of diagnosis during reference hospitalization

Source of diagnosis	Side	Restriction of spinal motion					Number known	Number unknown
		Right	Left	Bilateral	None	Total		
		HNP surgery at reference hospitalization						
Surgery	Right	19.3	6.8	44.3	29.5	99.9	176	5
Surgery	Left	7.0	20.0	38.9	34.1	100.0	185	10
Total*		12.9	13.5	42.2	31.4	100.0	379	16
		No HNP surgery at reference hospitalization						
Clinical	Right	17.2	7.6	39.9	35.4	100.1	198	11
Clinical	Left	5.5	17.4	40.6	36.5	100.0	219	20
Total†		11.4	13.7	39.5	35.5	100.1	651	77

*Percentages include 11 cases with a bilateral and 7 cases with unknown side of lesion diagnosed on HNP surgery. Restriction status was unknown for one other case.
†Percentages include 22 cases with a bilateral and 212 cases with unknown side of HNP lesion diagnosed clinically. Restriction status was unknown for 46 other cases.

Table 4-6. Probability of observed differences in rates of specified postural signs under hypothesis of no difference with status on other signs, by time of observation

Sign*	Time of observation							
	Reference hospitalization				Follow-up examination			
	Tilt	Paravertebral muscle spasm	Loss of lumbar lordosis	Restriction of motion	Tilt	Paravertebral muscle spasm	Loss of lumbar lordosis	Restriction of motion
Scoliosis	<.001†	—	—	<.01	—	<.001	<.005	<.001
Tilt		<.05	<.005	<.001		—	—	—
Paravertebral muscle spasm			<.001	<.001			<.001	<.001
Lumbar lordosis				<.001				<.001

*Status on these signs determined at time of observation.
†Presented are P values of ≤ .05 obtained on chi-square tests of significance. The − sign indicates P >.05 or insufficient observations. All significant differences are in the direction of higher rates with presence of other signs.

right, there generally was a corresponding restriction to the left. Table 4-3 shows the combinations of various restrictions of spinal motion when limitation of lateral flexion is grouped with limitation of rotation. Some restriction of spinal motion during the reference hospitalization was present in almost all patients. Limitation of lateral bending with or without limitation of rotation seldom occurred in the absence of limitation of forward flexion or extension.

The association of various restrictions of spinal motion with paravertebral muscle spasm and loss of lumbar lordosis is shown in Tables 4-4 and 4-6. Restricted spinal motion in all directions was more frequent when either of the other signs was present, and it was least frequent when both of the other signs were absent.

Table 4-7. Probability of observed differences in rates of specified postural signs under hypothesis of no difference with status on HNP surgery, by time of observation and time of surgery

	Time of observation			
	Reference hospitalization		Follow-up examination	
	Time of surgery		Time of surgery	
Sign*	Reference hospital	Follow-up period	Reference hospital	Follow-up period
Scoliosis	—†	—	—	—
Tilt	<.02	—	—	—
Paravertebral muscle spasm	<.02	—	—	—
Lumbar lordosis	<.001	—	—	<.005
Restriction of motion	—	—	—	<.001

*Status on these signs determined at time of observation.
†Presented are P values of ≤ .05 obtained on chi-square tests of significance. The − sign indicates P >.05. All significant differences are in direction of higher rate of positive findings in surgical group.

The extent of restricted spinal motion was not appreciably greater among patients who underwent HNP surgery during the reference hospitalization or the follow-up period than among the nonsurgical patients. The significance tests on these comparisons are summarized in Table 4-7. Over half (58.2%) of the patients who exhibited motor signs during the reference hospitalization had restrictions of spine motion in all directions, whereas only 48.4% of patients without motor signs had such restrictions. This difference, although not large, is significant (P <.05).

Table 4-5 indicates that there was a positive association between the side toward which spine motion was restricted and the side of the disc lesion (P <.001). In nonsurgical patients the observation of the side of the restriction may have affected the diagnosis of the side of the lesion. However, the same relationship is seen using the surgical diagnosis, which presumably is independent of clinical observation.

At follow-up examination, 86.6% of the patients had some restriction of spinal motion in each of the various directions. Limitations of flexion and extension of the lumbar spine were associated with each other, as well as with a limitation of lateral motion. Of the patients with either paravertebral muscle spasm, a loss of lumbar lordosis, or both, 95.1% had restricted lateral motion, often combined with reduced flexion and extension of the lumbar spine.

Patients who had not undergone surgery for HNP *in the follow-up period* had subsequent restriction of all spinal movements less frequently (21.2%) than patients operated on during that period (36.0%). However, restrictions of only lateral bending or rotation at follow-up were more frequent (23.9%) among patients not operated on during the follow-up period than in the other surgical groups (11.2%, P <.001). Surgery for HNP during the reference hospitalization was not associated with restriction of spinal motion at the follow-up examination. The significance of these relationships is summarized in Table 4-7. Patients with sensory signs at follow-up had a moderately but significantly greater frequency of restricted spinal movements in all directions (28.6%) than patients free of these signs (20.6%, P <.02).

Some restricted spinal motion appeared in almost all patients during the reference hospitalization. Evaluation of spinal movement adds less to the diagnosis of lumbar disc disease than do observations concerning spinal tilt and paravertebral muscle spasm.

Discussion

At the reference hospital examination, clinical signs related to spinal contour and the lumbar muscles were associated significantly with each other. This was especially true of the relationship between paravertebral muscle spasm, loss of lumbar lordosis, restricted spinal movement, and spinal tilt. The frequency of all these signs was higher during the reference hospitalization than at the follow-up examination: scoliosis, 52.9% and 14.0%; spinal tilt, 66.7% and 1.8%; muscle spasm, 71.6% and 11.9%; loss of lordosis, 57.7% and 30.3%; and restriction of spinal motion, 97.6% and 86.6%. Despite the reduced frequency of these signs, there seemed to be greater variability in the severity of the disease at the follow-up examination than during the reference hospitalization. Although, in general, patients showed a relative absence of postural signs at follow-up, those who remained disabled tended to exhibit multiple signs to a greater extent than during the reference hospitalization.

Patients who were operated on for HNP during the reference hospitalization tended to exhibit more postural signs at that time than patients not undergoing surgery, but there was no difference between these groups in the frequency of the postural signs detected at the follow-up examination. Patients with surgery *during*

Table 4-8. Percent of patients with weakness of specified muscle by side. Findings during reference hospitalization before reference date

Muscle	Right	Left
Dorsal flexors of foot	4.6	6.6
Plantar flexors of foot	1.8	2.7
Extensor hallucis longus	1.1	2.3
Quadriceps femoris	0.4	1.4
Other specified muscle	6.0	8.1
Unspecified weakness	6.8	10.4
No weakness	84.2	77.6
Number with known status	735	732
Number with unknown status	388	391

Table 4-9. Percent of patients with atrophy of specified muscle by side. Findings during reference hospitalization before reference date

Muscle	Right	Left
Buttock	3.8	4.1
Thigh	10.1	16.7
Calf	12.5	17.5
Other	0.5	0.4
Generalized or unspecified	2.7	3.2
Number with known status	821	822
Number with unknown status	302	301

the follow-up period, when seen later at the follow-up examination, tended to show loss of lordosis and restricted motion more often than those not operated on in this period.

NEUROLOGIC SIGNS
Motor signs

The records of the reference hospitalization were reviewed for evidence of weakness or atrophy of the muscles in the legs. The anatomic site of the weakness was noted, if mentioned. Weakness of leg muscles was recorded for 38.6% of the admissions, atrophy for 49.4%, and either or both of these motor signs for 63.2%.

During the reference hospitalization, weakness of a specific muscle was not a common finding, but unspecified motor weakness was more often recorded, as indicated in Table 4-8. Weakness was noted somewhat more frequently in the left than in the right leg. On the specific muscle tests, the extensor hallucis longus was weak more commonly than the quadriceps femoris. Atrophy also occurred more commonly in the left leg for most muscle groups and involved principally the thigh and calf muscles (Table 4-9). Almost two thirds (64.1%) of patients with muscle weakness had muscle atrophy; in patients without weakness, muscle atrophy occurred in 40.3%. Decreased tendon reflexes at the knee and ankle were associated with a somewhat higher frequency of atrophy in the legs (52.3%) than were normal reflexes (37.7%). The frequency of motor signs noted during the reference hospitalization did not vary appreciably with HNP surgery during either the reference hospitalization or the follow-up period. The statistical significance of the relationship of motor signs with sensory and reflex changes and with surgical status is given, respectively, in Tables 4-15 and 4-16.

At the follow-up examination, 70.5% of the patients had some motor signs, 35.5% had muscle weakness, and 58.4% had muscle atrophy. These percentages are similar to the rates with which motor signs were found during the reference hospitalization; thus these signs appear to persist in patients with lumbar disc disease.

At the follow-up examination, muscle weakness was found more frequently (50.7%) among those with HNP surgery in the follow-up period than among those not operated on during that time (32.2%). No significant difference in the frequency of motor signs at follow-up was found with surgical status during the reference hospitalization (Table 4-16). There was a strong positive association between the motor and the other neurologic signs (Table 4-15). Among patients with muscle weakness, 65.9%, and among patients free of muscle weakness, 54.3% had muscle atrophy.

Motor signs were a fairly frequent finding in patients with HNP. They persisted and apparently were not alleviated by surgery. This observation agrees with previous reports of the persistence of motor signs in patients relieved of pain and points to the possible significance of motor signs in determining disability.

Weakness was observed more often in the extensor hallucis longus muscle than in the quadriceps femoris, probably because minor degrees of weakness are more easily detected in the former. The finding of atrophy in almost two thirds of patients with muscle weakness agrees with earlier reports. Of uncertain value is the observation of atrophy in the absence of weakness. Although minor degrees of weakness may escape detection, this explanation is unsatisfactory. Perhaps

Table 4-10. Percent with decreased sensation in legs by site or dermatome level of lumbar disc lesion and by side. Findings during reference hospitalization prior to reference date

Site or dermatome	Right	Left
Anterior thigh or medial leg to ankle	0.8	0.8
Anterolateral thigh or anteromedial leg through big toe	4.4	5.5
Lateral thigh, anterolateral leg, top and sole of foot, toes 2, 3, 4	18.0	23.4
Posterolateral thigh, leg, foot, fifth toe	11.6	12.8
Stated as L3	1.0	1.9
Stated as L4	3.2	3.6
Stated as L5	7.9	11.3
Stated as S1	10.2	13.6
Other sensory change	6.6	9.8
Normal sensation	66.3	57.4
Total	100.0	100.0
Number with known status	964	981

muscle asymmetry due to unrelated causes was mistakenly attributed to an HNP, but this should not occur often. We cannot adequately explain the observation of atrophy without weakness in these data.

Sensory signs

Altered sensory function during the reference hospitalization was found in 69.0% of the patients, and hypesthesia was the most common finding occurring in 67.0%. Another 1.9% of the patients showed hyperesthesia. The left leg was involved somewhat more frequently than the right. Table 4-10 gives the frequency with which the various sensory deficits were observed. The records of the reference hospitalization revealed that involvement of the L5 dermatome was diagnosed in 28 patients, of whom 39.3% showed, at operation, localization to the L4-L5 level, 42.9% to L5-S1, and 10.7% to both levels. Conversely, there were 29 surgically confirmed findings at L4-L5, of which 72.4% were correctly inferred preoperatively. There were 41 patients with sensory changes involving the S1 dermatome for whom surgical findings were known. Of these, 65.9% had a surgically diagnosed lesion at L5-S1, and another 9.8% had lesions at both L4-L5 and L5-S1. Conversely, preoperative localization was correct in 80.0% of the L5-S1 lesions diagnosed surgically. Patients with changes of ankle and knee reflexes had associated sensory loss in 69.8%, whereas only 51.5% of those with normal reflexes had such changes. Operative status of the patient was not related to the presence of sensory signs at the reference hospitalization. The statistical significance of the relationship of sensory signs to other neurologic signs and to surgical status is shown in Tables 4-15 and 4-16.

At the follow-up examination, 50.7% had various sensory changes in either or both legs. Most of these changes were sensory deficits that occurred in 49.0%. The observations were obtained either from a specific evaluation of the dermatome level by the examining physician or from a drawing indicating the location of the sensory change. The distribution of lesions determined from these sources is shown in Table 4-11. The preferential involvement of the left leg over the right at the

Table 4-11. Percent distribution of dermatome lesions as inferred at follow-up examination from sensory deficits, by source of information and side

Dermatome	Physician's evaluation		Drawing	
	Right	Left	Right	Left
No decreased sensation	77.6	71.4	75.2	70.1
L4 only	0.7	1.7	0.3	0.8
L5 only	5.5	6.3	4.4	5.3
S1 only	6.6	7.1	4.0	4.5
L5 and S1, any	5.1	8.2	9.9	11.2
L5 with other multiple*	1.1	0.9	2.5	1.9
S1 with other multiple*	0.5	0.8	0.7	0.7
Other	2.8	3.5	3.1	5.5
Total	99.9	99.9	100.1	100.0
Number with known status	741	745	749	749
Number with unknown status	48	44	40	40

*Excluding combinations with L5 and S1, which are included above.

follow-up examination can also be seen. The frequency of involvement at the L5 level is similar to that at the S1 level. There were 39 patients with surgery at the reference hospitalization who had a sensory deficit at the follow-up examination from which the level of the disc was diagnosed at L4-L5. Among these 39 patients, 46.2% had a surgically confirmed lesion at the L4-L5 level and 7.7% at both L4-L5 and L5-S1. At follow-up the clinical diagnosis of the level of lesion at L4-L5 from the location of sensory change was correct in 82.1% of the lesions diagnosed at that level on surgery during the reference hospitalization. Of 32 patients with a lesion diagnosed on the follow-up examination at L5-S1, 65.6% had surgical verification at the L5-S1 level, and 15.6% at both the L4-L5 and the L5-S1 levels. When sensory signs were employed for a clinical diagnosis of level of HNP at follow-up, this procedure detected 58.2% of the L5-S1 lesions diagnosed on surgery at the reference hospitalization.

At the follow-up examination sensory deficit did not occur appreciably more often among patients operated on for HNP during the reference hospitalization (51.2%) compared with those not operated on (46.0%) at that time. However, patients operated on for HNP during the follow-up period had a higher frequency of sensory deficit (60.5%) than those not operated on in this period (45.6%). Results of statistical tests are summarized in Tables 4-15 and 4-16.

Sensory signs have been considered unreliable as a means of localizing the level of disc involvement, and observations in the present study are in accord. Like motor signs, sensory signs were found frequently in the 20-year follow-up examination of patients with a prior diagnosis of HNP; and also like motor signs, sensory signs were not significantly more frequent in patients who had undergone operation at the reference hospitalization.

Reflex signs

During the reference hospitalization, the ankle jerk was absent more often than the knee jerk and absent slightly more often in the left leg (Table 4-12). Reflexes were normal in 156 men, increased in 54, decreased or absent in 663, a combination

Table 4-12. Percent distribution of tendon reflex status by site and side. Findings during reference hospitalization before reference date

Tendon reflex status	Ankle		Knee	
	Right	Left	Right	Left
Normal	43.3	39.5	59.8	55.7
Increased	9.3	8.9	16.9	17.9
Reduced	20.7	24.7	18.2	20.3
Absent	23.7	22.7	2.9	2.7
Increased and decreased or absent	3.0	4.2	2.2	3.4
Total	100.0	100.0	100.0	100.0
Number with known status	1,073	1,079	1,048	1,055
Number with unknown status	50	44	75	68

Table 4-13. Percent distribution of tendon reflex status by site and side. Findings at follow-up examination

Tendon reflex status	Ankle		Knee	
	Right	Left	Right	Left
Normal	55.0	52.8	79.8	80.2
Increased	2.0	1.5	4.1	4.1
Reduced	20.5	21.4	15.1	14.4
Absent	22.4	24.2	1.0	1.3
Total	99.9	99.9	100.0	100.0
Number with known status	784	784	782	783
Number with unknown status	339	339	341	340

Table 4-14. Number of patients by strength of dorsiflexor muscle and ankle reflex status and side. Findings during reference hospitalization before the reference date

Ankle reflex status	Weak dorsiflexor			Normal dorsiflex*	Total known status	Unknown status
	Bilateral	Right	Left			
Bilateral decreased	1	9	8	120	138	69
Right only decreased	0	20	1	176	197	104
Left only decreased	0	1	27	207	235	115
Neither decreased nor absent	0	3	11	138	152	85
Unknown status	0	0	0	11	11	17
Total	1	33	47	652	733	390

*Includes weakness of other leg muscles not combined with dorsiflexor weakness.

of increased and decreased or absent at the different sites in 236, and unknown in 14. They were decreased or absent at either the knee or the ankle in one or both legs in 81.1% of the patients. During the reference hospitalization, reflex changes were moderately associated with muscle weakness and strongly associated with muscle atrophy (Table 4-15). There was no significant association with surgical status (Table 4-16).

The ankle jerk was absent or reduced in 82.9% of the patients with a pre-operative diagnosis of an L5-S1 lesion and in only 69.1% in those with a diagnosis of L4-L5 (P <.001). A similar association is observed when only the surgical diagnosis of level is used. The relationship between the ankle reflex changes and the level of disc lesion appears somewhat stronger than that established for sensory deficits, but because of the limited numbers in this analysis, reflex signs cannot be shown to provide any more effective means of diagnosing level than is provided by sensory signs.

At the follow-up examination, the ankle reflex was absent in more than one fourth of the patients, whereas the knee reflex was absent in only a few (Table 4-13). The frequency of a decreased reflex was equal for the two legs. Decreased or absent reflexes in either or both legs were noted in 68.3%. Hyperactive reflexes were rarely found at the follow-up examination, although they often occurred in combination with decreased reflexes during the reference hospitalization (21.3% of the admissions). Patients operated on at the reference hospitalization had decreased or absent reflexes at the follow-up examination more often (77.7%) than did those without HNP surgery (62.2%). Patients operated on in the follow-up period also had a higher rate of hypoactive reflexes (76.0%) compared with those not operated during that time (66.4%).

As in other studies, diminution or loss of the ankle jerk was somewhat corre-lated with HNP at the L5-S1 level. The persistence of hypoactive or absent reflexes also followed general experience. Of uncertain significance was the frequent finding of hyperactive reflexes during the reference hospitalization. In these data hyper-active reflexes of the ankle cannot be explained by weakness of antagonistic muscle groups, that is, of 3 patients with increased reflexes on the right and of 7 patients with increased reflexes on the left, only 1 and 3, respectively, had weak dorsiflexors on the corresponding side. However, Table 4-14 indicates that during the reference hospitalization there was a strong relationship (P <.001) between decreased reflexes and weakness of the dorsiflexor muscles on the affected side. There was no relationship between the recorded strength of the quadriceps femoris and increased knee reflexes, and a slight tendency to weakness with decreased reflexes.

Straight leg raising (SLR)

During the reference hospitalization, information on the outcome of the straight leg raising (SLR) test was available for 1,048 of the patients, and of these patients 96.4% had abnormal findings. Included as indications of a positive SLR test were statements in the records of the reference hospitalization regarding positive Lasègue test, crossed Lasègue test, and positive Kernig test. The left leg was involved only slightly more frequently than the right. At less than 30 degrees the test was posi-tive on the right in 17.4% and on the left in 18.4%. Limitation from 31 degrees to 70 degrees occurred in the right leg in 27.0% and in the left leg in 28.8%. Of the patients with no HNP surgery during the reference hospitalization, 95.1% had a positive SLR test, whereas 97.6% of the patients with HNP operations during the reference hospitalization had a positive SLR test before surgery. The difference is not significant. However, the so-called crossed Lasègue sign was positive for 18.7% of the patients with HNP surgery during the reference hospitalization and for only 9.5% of those without such surgery (P <.001).

Table 4-15. Probability of observed differences in rates of specified neurologic signs under hypothesis of no difference with status on other signs, by time of observation

| | Time of observation | | | | | |
| | Reference hospitalization | | | Follow-up examination | | |
Sign*	Muscle atrophy	Decreased sensation	Reflex change	Muscle atrophy	Decreased sensation	Reflex change
Muscle weakness	<.001†	<.001	—	<.005	<.001	<.001
Muscle atrophy		—	≃.05		<.001	<.05
Decreased sensation			<.001			<.001

*Status on these signs determined at time of observation.
†Presented are P values of ≤ .05 obtained on chi-square tests of significance. The − sign indicates P >.05 or insufficient observations. All significant differences are in the direction of higher rates with presence of other sign.

Table 4-16. Probability of observed differences in rates of specified neurologic signs under hypothesis of no difference with status on HNP surgery, by time of observation and time of surgery

	Time of observation			
	Reference hospitalization		Follow-up examination	
	Time of surgery		Time of surgery	
Sign*	Reference hospital	Follow-up period	Reference hospital	Follow-up period
Muscle weakness	—†	—	—	<.001
Muscle atrophy	—	—	—	—
Decreased sensation	—	—	—	<.005
Reflex change	—	—	<.001	<.05

*Status on these signs determined at time of observation.
†Presented are P values of ≤ .05 obtained on chi-square tests of significance. The − sign indicates P >.05. All significant differences are in direction of higher rate of positive findings in surgical group.

Abnormal SLR results were found for either or both legs at follow-up in 38.6% of patients tested. Among the patients whose SLR values were determined at follow-up, no meaningful differences in the frequency of positive findings were associated with surgical status. Among 244 patients with simultaneous motor, sensory, and reflex signs at follow-up, 49.2% also had abnormal SLR findings. Among the remaining 492 patients with recorded observations of both SLR and neurologic signs, 33.5% had abnormal SLR findings (P <.001). Thus at the follow-up examination the SLR test was shown to be associated significantly with the presence of neurologic signs.

The quite high frequency of an abnormal SLR sign in this sample of patients with a hospitalization for HNP was to be expected because of the high rates of other signs. Although the frequency of abnormal SLR signs at the reference hospitalization was no different between surgical and nonsurgical groups, positive findings on the crossed Lasègue test were significantly related to the likelihood of HNP surgery.

During the follow-up period positive findings on the SLR test subsided to a great extent. At the follow-up examination almost two thirds of the patients had normal results; however, positive findings were strongly associated with the presence of other neurologic signs. This study failed to establish the value of a positive

SLR test in predicting the outcome of surgical and nonsurgical treatment. It confirms the observations reported by others that few patients with HNP may be normal in SLR tests and that many patients with positive results in SLR tests will recover without operation.

Jugular compression test

The jugular compression test was positive in 42.6% of the 612 patients for whom results were recorded during the reference hospitalization. Patients without HNP surgery had a lower frequency of positive findings (37.8%) during the reference hospitalization than patients operated on for HNP had before surgery (48.7%, P <.01).

At follow-up, the frequency of positive tests was reduced to 3.1%. Among the 470 nonsurgical patients, 2.8%, and among the 295 surgical patients whose status on the test was determined, 3.7% were positive. The difference is not significant. No significant association existed between a positive jugular compression test and the other neurologic signs at follow-up.

Other tests

There were 88 men with a positive Patrick test, 38 with a positive Gaenslen test, 16 with a positive Ely test, and 92 with positive findings on various other tests. A positive finding on one of these tests was generally associated with positive findings on one or more of the others.

Discussion

Motor, sensory, and reflex signs were associated with each other during the reference hospitalization and at the follow-up examination. The percentage of motor signs was similar during the reference hospitalization (63.2%) and at follow-up (70.5%); however, muscle atrophy predominated at the latter examination. Sensory defects were observed in 69.0% of men during reference hospitalization and in 50.7% at follow-up. Decreased ankle and knee reflexes were noted in 81.1% at the reference hospitalization and in 68.3% at follow-up. The frequencies of positive SLR findings at those times were 96.4% and 38.6%, respectively, and for the jugular compression test, 42.6% and 3.1%.

A slightly greater frequency of neurologic signs observed during the reference hospitalization in the surgical patients was not statistically significant. Later, at the follow-up examination, the neurologic signs generally were most frequent among patients operated on during the follow-up period, less frequent among patients operated on only during the reference hospitalization, and least frequent among those who were never operated on.

SUMMARY

The various objective signs of lumbar disc disease, observed before surgery or within 90 days of admission for lumbar HNP to the first Army (reference) hospital, were grouped to reflect either postural or neurologic mechanisms. In general, for both types of signs the frequency of abnormal findings was initially high, and almost all patients exhibited various combinations of signs. Twenty years after the first hospital admission for HNP, in this sample of patients, there was an appreciable decrease in the frequency of the postural signs and of positive findings on the SLR and jugular compression tests. Of greatest significance among the postural signs is paravertebral muscle spasm, which occurs commonly with the other postural alterations. Patients selected for HNP surgery at the reference hospital had a higher incidence of spasm, which, because of its objective nature and ease of observation, can be considered a reliable index of a symptomatic lumbar HNP. Paravertebral muscle spasm was a relatively infrequent finding 20 years later; but if it was present, it tended to persist with the other postural and neurologic signs.

Postural alterations, such as loss of lumbar lordosis, occurred in the initial phases of the disease in more than half the patients. About one third of the patients did not have normal lumbar lordosis at the 20-year examination, and it was usually associated with some degree of restricted spinal motion or other signs.

Among the neurologic signs found during the reference hospitalization, the motor signs, consisting of weakness and atrophy of the muscles in the involved leg, were prominent. Atrophy, involving primarily thigh and calf muscles, was noted more often in the left leg than in the right. Almost half the patients were found to have weakness of the leg muscles during the reference hospitalization, and it was associated with a higher prevalence of decreased sensation. The motor signs persisted 20 years later, regardless of whether surgery had been done. Muscle weakness could be considered a fairly reliable index to physical disability in persons with HNP. A strong association between motor and other neurologic signs was noted at the 20-year follow-up examination.

Initially, hypesthesia was the most common sensory change; only an occasional patient exhibited hyperesthesia. The sensory deficit was more common in the left leg, as were the initial pain and the motor symptoms. In a fairly high percentage of patients the sensory change occurred over the specific dermatome corresponding to the level of the disc involved. About 85% of the patients with a specific sensory loss also had reductions in their tendon reflexes at the ankle or knee. Twenty years later, at the follow-up examination, half the patients still exhibited sensory deficits with the left leg preference still present. The sensory dermatome involvement at the follow-up examination also corresponded fairly well with the original disc level diagnosed surgically during the reference hospitalization.

Reflex signs were found frequently during the reference hospitalization. They occurred more often in the left leg than in the right and were strongly associated with sensory deficit. The ankle jerk was absent more often than the knee jerk and was associated with a disc localized at the L5-S1 level. Neither the reflex signs nor the sensory signs provide an accurate means of localizing the level of the lesion clinically. Twenty years later, the ankle jerk was still often absent, and alterations in the reflexes were noted to be slightly more frequent in the surgical patients.

The straight leg raising sign has always been considered to indicate sciatic nerve irritation and to be often associated with HNP. Almost all patients exhibited this sign during the reference hospitalization. During that hospitalization, surgery for HNP was carried out more frequently among patients with a positive *crossed* straight leg raising sign than among those without crossed findings. The test, evaluated 20 years later, showed a rather significant association with the presence of other neurologic signs, but did not distinguish between surgical and nonsurgical patients.

The jugular compression test was positive in slightly less than half the patients in the initial evaluation, but 20 years later it was found in only a few, and when it was present, it showed no association with other neurologic signs.

Viewed only in terms of results, the surgical group appeared to fare no better than the group that did not undergo operation. However, since the surgical group was characterized by failure to improve with conservative treatment, their disease may have been different from or more severe than the disease of patients who responded to nonsurgical measures. On the other hand, the persistence of abnormal findings might be interpreted as a reason for reexamining indications for surgical versus nonsurgical treatment.

CHAPTER 5

EVALUATION OF SURGICAL AND CONSERVATIVE THERAPY OF LUMBAR DISC LESIONS

HUBERT L. ROSOMOFF

A variety of circumstances appear to have influenced the modes of therapy and, therefore, the analysis of this study group of 1,123 subjects. It was shown in the preceding chapters that surgical patients differ in several important respects from those treated conservatively. Although it has been possible to evaluate disability at the time of the follow-up examination by the same statistical techniques in all patients, regardless of treatment experience, differences between surgical and non-surgical patients are difficult to interpret because their illness and history before the reference hospitalization were not quite comparable, and Army management policies and criteria affected selection of therapeutic modes. Biases that statistical methods are unable to exclude may have been introduced. In this chapter we delineate the modes of management of lumbar disc lesions in the Army hospitals, specify the known differences between surgical and nonsurgical patients, and attempt to interpret the results in the light of present-day management of lumbar disc disease.

CONSERVATIVE THERAPY

The various measures used in conservative therapy during the reference hospitalization are listed in Table 5-1. Physical therapy and bed rest were the primary modalities, followed in decreasing order by leg or other traction, procaine and other anesthetic injections, braces or casts, and other miscellanea. The table includes methods applied to nonsurgical patients and applied before surgical intervention, but the data are not complete. The absence of a statement in the record may not always mean that the treatment was not applied. For example, the records of 544 patients did not indicate whether bed rest was prescribed, and the records of 449 did not indicate the number of days of bed rest. There were also 70 patients for whom an operation was advised but who refused; and 6 patients were judged to be surgical candidates but were excluded because of a psychiatric disease. In the sample of 1,123 men, 400 (35.6%) eventually came to surgery during the reference hospitalization, and in 395 (35.2%) of these the surgery was for HNP. Another 101 of the original nonsurgical patients underwent an operation for HNP during the follow-up period. Thus 496 (44.2%) of the entire group had surgical intervention for HNP.

Conservative management resulted in complete relief of symptoms in only 3.1% of the 948 patients whose treatment results were recorded. The largest number (64.1%) obtained partial or temporary relief; and 32.8% had no relief. In another 175 patients the extent of benefit could not be determined from the

Table 5-1. Percent distribution of type of conservative therapy during reference hospitalization among 875 cases on whom any information was available*

Therapy	Percent	Number
None	1.6	14
Bed rest, full or part time	63.2	553
Lumbosacral belt, etc.	7.3	64
Physiotherapy	72.5	634
Postural exercises	8.2	72
Manipulation of back	4.2	37
Leg or other traction	16.2	142
Procaine injection, etc.	13.3	116
Brace or body cast	10.2	89
Other specified	7.4	65

*Including information on surgical cases before the date of surgery.

record. Among the 311 failures (32.8%) 172 patients were treated later with surgery. In each surgical status group, patients treated with braces or casts seemed to have derived some benefit from them.

It has not been possible to evaluate fully the various forms of conservative therapy. Apparently some mode of treatment was applied in almost every patient, especially when surgical intervention was not judged necessary or was interdicted by policy. If conservative therapy was successful, surgical intervention was less likely. In the surgical group, temporary relief of symptoms through conservative therapy was reported for 43.2% of the patients; in the conservatively treated group 74.0% obtained temporary, and 4.5% obtained complete, relief of symptoms (P < .001). However, it appears that the factors leading to the selection of patients for surgery were fairly complex. An analysis of the data demonstrates no association between directed conservative therapy (defined as bed rest of 8 days or more, traction, physical therapy, manipulation, and brace or body cast) and the neurologic signs. But when postural signs—such as loss of lordosis, paravertebral muscle spasm, etc.—or a positive straight leg raising test were present, directed conservative management was found to be employed more commonly. It is not altogether certain that conservative management was more likely to be directed if the patient exhibited postural signs, as opposed to neurologic signs. Postural signs may have been more likely to be detected or recorded when conservative treatment was prescribed specifically.

SURGICAL THERAPY

Among the 400 patients who underwent surgery during the reference hospitalization, 395 had an operation for a herniated lumbar disc. The other 5 patients were listed as having had explorations, rhizotomy, or nerve root decompression. Of the 395 men, 14.7% had surgery for HNP again during the follow-up period, either in the VA system or in private hospitals. Of the 728 patients who did not have an operation for herniated lumbar disc during the reference hospitalization, 13.9% also eventually came to surgery. As with conservative treatment modes, the type of operation to be performed during the reference hospitalization was not standardized according to Army protocol; this was left to the preference of the surgeon. The usual surgical technique at that time was the removal of the extruded disc fragment or of the degenerated fragments within the disc space without an

Table 5-2. Percent and number of patients by type of procedure on HNP surgery during reference hospitalization and during follow-up

Type of procedure	Reference hospital		Follow-up	
	Percent	Number*	Percent	Number†
Partial laminectomy	66.1	261	84.9	135
Total, bilateral laminectomy	1.8	7	7.5	12
Interlaminar removal, no bone removed	28.4	112	13.8	22
Fusion	3.0	12	23.9	38
Decompression of nerve root (bone removed over root)	4.1	16	6.3	10
Unilateral procedure	92.7	366	82.4	131
Bilateral procedure	4.8	19	11.3	18
Multiple interspace	31.4	124	52.2	83
Other	6.1	24	10.1	16
Total with HNP surgery	100.0	395	100.0	159

*On first operation for HNP at reference hospital.
†Multiple operations with different types of surgery counted once under each type.

effort to carry out an extensive removal of intervertebral disc material. Table 5-2 indicates that, regardless of the time of surgery, partial laminectomy was the most frequent procedure followed by interlaminar removal. Total bilateral laminectomy during the reference hospitalization was rare. It was somewhat more common during the follow-up period, but it still accounted for only 7.5% of the 159 operations performed in that interval.

Explorations of multiple interspaces were done on about one third of the surgical patients during the reference hospitalization and on about one half of those operated on during follow-up. Fusion of vertebrae during the reference hospitalization was exceptional, but it was carried out in almost one fourth of the men with HNP surgery during the follow-up period. The frequency of fusion during follow-up was 23.8% among the 101 patients with no HNP surgery during the reference hospitalization and 24.1% among the 58 patients with HNP surgery both during the reference hospitalization and subsequently. As a result of operative intervention at the reference hospitalization, there were eight wound infections designated as moderate or severe, but no instances of paraplegia were recorded. After HNP surgery at the reference hospital, 5.1% of the patients reported no residual pain, 11.6% reported leg pain only, 18.0% reported back pain only, and 52.2% reported both leg and back pain.

Both during the reference hospitalization and during the follow-up period, the pathologic lesion found on HNP surgery was generally described as a herniation or a protrusion, as indicated in Table 5-3. The designation of free fragment or extrusion was fairly common, and 2 patients were said to have a "concealed" disc on surgery at the reference hospital. Table 5-4 shows that the lesion was diagnosed more often at the L5-S1 level than at the L4-L5 level on reference hospital surgery, but the diagnoses from HNP surgery during follow-up were evenly divided between these two levels. Lesions in more than one interspace were diagnosed in 7.6% of the HNP operations done during the reference hospitalization and in 17.6% of the HNP operations done during the follow-up period. The latter percentage in-

Table 5-3. Percent and number of cases with specified operative findings during reference hospitalization and during follow-up

Operative findings	Reference hospital		Follow-up	
	Percent	Number*	Percent	Number*
Herniated nucleus, protrusion	81.5	322	82.4	131
Free fragment, extrusion	17.5	69	21.4	34
Concealed disc, disc "bulges on flexion"	0.5	2	0	0
Midline protrusion	6.6	26	6.3	10
Undue vertical mobility, unstable joint	1.5	6	11.9	19
Thickened or hypertrophic ligamentum flavum	12.4	49	6.9	11
Excessive extradural veins	4.6	18	3.1	5
Other	24.6	97	53.5	85
Number with HNP surgery	100.0	395	100.0	159

*Some patients counted in more than one category of operative findings.

Table 5-4. Percent and number of location of operative findings on HNP surgery during reference hospitalization and during follow-up

Location	Reference hospital		Follow-up	
	Percent	Number	Percent	Number
L3–L4 only	1.3	5	3.1	5
L4–L5 only	32.7	129	39.6	63
L5–S1 only	55.4	219	35.2	56
L3–L4 and L4–L5	1.0	4	0.6	1
L4–L5 and L5–S1	6.6	26	17.0	27
Other	2.8	11	3.8	6
Unknown	0.3	1	0.6	1
Right	45.8	181	39.6	63
Left	49.4	195	48.4	77
Bilateral	3.0	12	7.5	12
Total	100.0	395	100.0	159

cludes several patients with diagnoses at a different single level obtained from repeated operations.

COMPARISON OF SURGICAL AND CONSERVATIVE THERAPY AT THE REFERENCE HOSPITAL

A direct comparison of treatment results is not appropriate because of the possible bias in selection for treatment during the reference hospitalization cited earlier. However, it is of interest to evaluate the differences between the surgical and the nonsurgical groups to determine how the initial selection might affect subsequent findings. Some of these data were presented in Chapter 2. In the surgical group the mean number of prior service hospital admissions for back or leg complaints (not leading to an HNP diagnosis) was 0.51, whereas in the nonsurgical group it was 0.57—a small and not significant difference. Patients who underwent HNP surgery during the reference hospitalization were more likely to receive VA compensation for HNP disability or a disability pension 1 year after separation from service (97.2%) than were nonsurgical patients (90.9%, P <.001). At the cutoff date of follow-up observations, 93.9% of the surgical patients and 80.5% of the nonsurgical patients were still being compensated or pensioned for HNP disability (P <.001). The mean age at the reference hospital admission of the surgical patients was 29.0 years, compared with 30.0 years among those treated conservatively—a moderate but significant (P <.01) difference. In the surgical group, at the military service induction examination, 5.3% were found to have objective signs pertaining to the back or the legs, compared with 9.5% in the non-

Table 5-5. Percent with objective back or leg signs noted on induction physical examination and total number by duration of leg pain before reference hospitalization and by surgical status during reference hospitalization

Duration of leg pain (months)	HNP surgery		No HNP surgery		Total	
	Percent with signs	Total* number	Percent with signs	Total* number	Percent with signs	Total* number
≤ 2	4.1	146	4.6	241	4.4	387
3–11	3.9	128	6.8	161	5.5	289
12+	8.9	112	15.6	294	13.8	406
Unknown	0.0	7	3.7	27	2.9	34
Total	5.3	393	9.5	723	8.1	1,116

*Status with respect to back and leg signs was unknown for 2 cases in the group with HNP surgery and for 5 cases in the group without HNP surgery.

Table 5-6. Percent of patients with specified signs or symptoms by time of observation and surgical status during reference hospitalization

Signs or symptoms at time of observation	Time of observation					
	Reference hospitalization*			Follow-up examination		
	Surgery for HNP	No surgery for HNP	Significance of difference†	Surgery for HNP	No surgery for HNP	Significance of difference†
Postural						
Lumbar scoliosis	56.3	50.6	—	13.6	14.5	—
Spinal tilt	72.4	63.5	<.02	1.6	1.9	—
Paravertebral muscle spasm	76.5	68.8	<.02	13.0	11.2	—
Loss of lumbar lordosis	65.9	52.6	<.001	31.3	29.7	—
Restricted motion of spine (in all directions)	52.2	52.4	—	23.5	25.1	—
Localized percussion, positive	66.2	58.4	—	32.0	32.1	—
Localized tenderness	(Not recorded consistently)			42.4	41.6	—
Neurologic						
Weakness of leg muscles	40.2	37.7	—	38.5	33.3	—
Atrophy of leg muscles	53.4	47.0	—	55.7	60.1	—
Decreased sensation in legs	66.7	67.3	—	51.2	46.0	—
Decreased reflexes in legs	83.0	80.0	—	77.7	62.2	<.001
Straight leg raising test, positive	97.6	95.1	—	39.5	38.1	—
Back pain with sciatica	96.9	95.9	—	47.7	58.0	<.005

*Observed before HNP surgery if any was performed.
†Presented are P values of ≤.05 obtained on chi-square tests of significance. The — sign indicates P >.05.

surgical group (P <.02). Moreover, the frequency of the defects was significantly related to the duration of leg pain, before the reference hospitalization, as shown in Table 5-5 (P <.001). In Chapter 3 we showed that HNP surgery was more frequent among patients with back pain of shorter duration. It is, therefore, likely that the nonsurgical group included a somewhat greater proportion of older, long-term chronic patients than the group who underwent surgery during the reference hospitalization.

A systematic comparison of clinical findings by surgical status is shown in Table 5-6. In the surgical group there were significantly greater frequencies during the reference hospitalization of spinal tilt, paravertebral muscle spasm, and loss of lumbar lordosis than in the nonsurgical group. Differences with respect to neurologic signs observed during the reference hospitalization were slight. Moreover, almost all patients had either motor or sensory signs or reflex signs. When the presence of all these signs is required before a case is classified as positive, again no significant difference is evident between the surgical and nonsurgical cases. This may have occurred because:

1. In fact, only postural signs were considered in selecting cases for surgery.
2. The clinical examination for postural signs on cases scheduled for surgery was more critical.
3. The findings of postural signs on cases scheduled for surgery were detailed in the records more precisely.
4. There was a combination of these factors.

Table 5-6 also shows that at the follow-up examination, except for decreased reflexes, the surgical patients had almost no preponderance of objective signs, compared with the nonsurgical patients. The surgical patients did report less sciatic pain and a significantly greater frequency of decreased reflexes at follow-up. For both surgical status groups the frequency of muscle atrophy was higher at follow-up than at the initial examination. Thus no appreciable differences in clinically detectable disability at the follow-up examination were associated with surgical status at the reference hospitalization. However, the rate of hospital readmissions for back or leg symptoms during the follow-up period was slightly higher among those with HNP surgery at the reference hospitalization (44.9%) than among nonsurgical patients (37.9%, P <.05).

Specific analysis of frequency of clinical signs at the follow-up examination by their presence during the reference hospitalization is presented in Chapter 6 and will help to clarify some of these relationships. Differences between surgical groups evaluated by items on occupation, the examiner's functional rating, and the VA compensation rating will also be presented in Chapter 6 in detail. In summary, no significant difference in the use of the back at follow-up was associated with surgical status. It is easy to understand why a VA compensation rating would be higher among surgical patients with a scar on the back, and it is therefore important to note that the more objective examiner's functional impression of the follow-up examination showed less bias, with almost equal mean values in the two surgical groups.

DISCUSSION

If the data presented are accepted without a critical evaluation, there seems to be no clear difference in the results of treatment of HNP between conservative and surgical modes. The nonsurgically oriented reader might interpret the data as indicating that conservative treatment is as good as surgery if the patient can persist long enough with the former method. Why operate if there is no difference in the outcome and the risk of having to do a subsequent operation is unaffected by whether the earlier surgery has been carried out? This argument is hard to refute from the data at hand until an explanation is sought in the clinical management of the patients. Then, the surgeon will just as easily come to the conclusion that the results of treatment for both groups are just as bad. This attitude may be based on the therapeutic experience of the last three decades, not available or utilized by the Army Medical Corps in the era under review.

It is important to reiterate the bias introduced by Army treatment policy. The methods of management of the lumbar herniated nucleus pulposus that had been used in civilian medical practice were found early not to be applicable in the military. Policies evolved partly in response to Army manpower needs, rather than representing preferred treatment modes. The likely results of these policies were prolonged attempts at conservative management, less early referral, and more stringent justifications for surgery. Furthermore, early failures were produced, paradoxically, by an otherwise excellent program of physical therapy, which, however, proved ill-adapted to patients with low back disabilities. Most disc patients reacted unfavorably to the regimen, many requiring rehospitalization during service because of recurring symptomatology. It is probable that the existence of the program affected the selection of patients for surgery and the decision as to when in the course of treatment surgery should be carried out. The absence of reliable posttreatment records during the reference hospitalization with which to compare the follow-up data also represents a limitation on the ability to interpret treatment results. Without these data it is impossible to determine to what extent signs disappeared immediately postoperatively, to appear anew later and to persist until the time of the follow-up examination.

It is clear from treatises on the subject that the most dependable index of the successful treatment of lumbar nerve root compression, by any method, is the disappearance of leg pain, which was indeed less prevalent at follow-up in the surgical group. The relief of back pain is not as reliable, and the regression of postural and neurologic deficits, however desirable, is the least consistent of all. In these respects the present data are confirmatory.

Modern practice dictates an initial trial of bed rest plus analgesics, muscle relaxants, and physiotherapy for a period of 10 days to 2 weeks for the herniated lumbar disc patient without overt bladder retention, or severe motor deficit. If an initial satisfactory response is obtained, as judged by decreased pain and regression of physical signs, conservative management is continued until the symptoms and signs abate completely or until it is seen that further treatment will fail to resolve the clinical problem entirely. The latter condition or an initial unsatisfactory response calls for the consideration of surgical intervention, and the total period from initiation of treatment to the choice of the final mode of therapy is usually within 2 to 6 weeks, or 8 weeks at the most. The conservative surgical techniques used with these patients may also affect the evaluation of surgical results.

It is apparent from Table 5-7 that decisions on surgery were long delayed in the present sample. More than 80% of the surgical patients were operated on after delays of 2 or 3 months. It seems plausible, then, that surgery, although still giving

Table 5-7. Percent distribution of time from reference hospital admission to surgery by type of conservative therapy before surgery among surgical patients

Months from admission to surgery	Directed conservative therapy	No directed conservative therapy	Total with surgery
0	1.7	6.3	3.5
1	11.6	20.9	15.3
2	17.4	21.5	19.0
3	18.2	13.9	16.5
4+	51.2	37.3	45.8
Total	100.1	99.9	100.1
Total number	242	158	400

Table 5-8. Percent with sciatica at follow-up examination by interval from reference hospital admission to HNP surgery and nature of preoperative management

Interval from admission to HNP surgery	Preoperative management		Total
	Directed conservative therapy	No directed conservative therapy*	
1–2 months	50.8	50.0	50.4
3 months	51.2	42.1	48.3
4 + months	60.0	67.4	62.3
No HNP surgery	63.6	68.7	65.1
Total	60.6	62.3	61.2

*Includes cases with nature of conservative therapy not recorded.

good relief from pain, failed to resolve neurologic deficits that by the time of intervention had become irreversible. Similarly, immobilization with conservative management, when prolonged, may well yield an increased number of patients with pain relief. However, this may be at the cost of a greater percentage with neurologic residua. Thus, at final evaluation, both treatment modes could produce a disproportionately higher number of patients with irreversible physical findings and, probably, less pain relief than could have been achieved by a judicious application of both therapies. This is attested to by the more than 30% of patients from both treatment groups who required further hospitalization after discharge from the service, almost half within a period of a year.

It is possible, therefore, that neither surgical nor conservative treatment gave its best predictable results, according to present standards; they may be equally bad. Although this interpretation seems plausible, the available data give it only limited empirical support. No significant differences can be demonstrated in an overall evaluation of disability with time from reference hospital admission to surgery. However, the frequency of sciatica at the follow-up examination is somewhat lower ($P < .05$) among surgical patients operated on during the first 3 months of the reference hospitalization than among those with surgery later in the reference hospitalization or among those with no surgery. These differences persist, regardless of the nature of conservative therapy before surgery, as indicated in Table 5-8. Because we are not dealing with a treatment experiment, even in this comparison, considerable selection may have taken place. The primary significance of these data, therefore, is not in an evaluation of treatments, but in an assessment of the extent to which symptoms subsided in each of the treatment groups over an extended period of follow-up.

SUMMARY

During the reference hospitalization 395 patients were treated surgically for HNP, whereas 723 were treated conservatively, and 5 had back surgery other than removal of disc. The surgical patients had, before surgery, somewhat greater frequencies of postural signs than patients treated conservatively, but no significant differences in the occurrence of neurologic signs have been noted with surgical status. Patients selected for surgery and those treated conservatively differed in other important respects, and this makes it impossible to compare treatment results directly. In the light of present management, attempts at conservative therapy seem to have been prolonged unduly before surgery was undertaken. Among the patients with HNP surgery during the reference hospitalization, 14.7% were operated on again for HNP during follow-up; among those without HNP surgery during the reference hospitalization, 13.9% had follow-up operations. Patients with HNP surgery during the reference hospitalization significantly less often had back pain with sciatica at the follow-up examination, and significantly more often had decreased reflexes of the knee or ankle as well as rehospitalization for disc symptoms during the follow-up period, compared with nonsurgical patients.

CHAPTER *6*

EVALUATION OF DISABILITY
FROM DISC DISEASE

JAMES E. NIXON and ZDENEK HRUBEC

In the last 10 to 15 years there has developed an increasing concern about the reliability of the physician as he conducts and evaluates the clinical examination. Our data have been obtained through such examinations, but by different methods at two separate points in time. The first set of observations was made under only fairly uniform conditions in the military setting, when a diagnosis of HNP was first applied, and the second was obtained more than 20 years later, when disability from the disease was evaluated according to a standard examination protocol using carefully formulated definitions. The unique contribution of the study is the standardized follow-up examination of a clearly defined group of disc patients on whom earlier baseline observations were available.

The sampling of the military experience made possible the definition of a representative group whose composition did not change throughout the period of follow-up. At the end of that period 70.3% of the patients could be examined. The generality of the follow-up findings may be assessed by comparing the characteristics of those examined with those not examined. In earlier sections there was some indication that the examined patients had somewhat higher rates of HNP surgery and of hospital readmission during the follow-up period. This difference may reflect administrative factors related to the availability of VA compensation, or it may be the result of differences in the severity of the disease between examined and not examined patients during the follow-up period or at the reference hospitalization. Table 6-1 indicates that during the reference hospitalization there were no appreciable differences in the frequency of neurologic and postural signs between patients whose status on the same signs was determined at the follow-up examination and those whose status was not known. The only statistically significant (P <.05), although slight, difference is in the frequency of loss of lumbar lordosis during the reference hospitalization. There was a tendency to examine the patients with more severe disability at follow-up, but the reference hospital clinical findings are comparable for those with and without follow-up examination data.

The original baseline observations were not made with any later study in mind, but they lend themselves to present application through the increased awareness of the Army neurosurgeons of the significance of the HNP syndrome in relation to military manpower needs, and of the need to document the onset of the disease in relation to any later compensation claims. For many patients a standard neurologic form (U.S. Army Form 55E) had been filled out during the reference hospitaliza-

Table 6-1. Percent of patients with positive findings on specified items during the reference hospitalization, by availability of follow-up examination data on specified item

Item	Examined and status known at follow-up		Not examined or status unknown at follow-up		Total	
	Percent positive	Total number*	Percent positive	Total number*	Percent positive	Total number*
Postural						
Lumbar scoliosis	54.6	504	48.5	198	52.8	702
Spinal tilt	68.4	509	62.2	193	66.7	702
Paravertebral muscle spasm	71.0	732	72.7	319	71.6	1,051
Loss of lumbar lordosis	60.0	732	52.4	319	57.7	1,051
Restricted spine motion	53.5	694	50.0	336	52.3	1,030
Neurologic						
Weakness of leg muscles	39.1	443	36.8	174	38.4	617
Atrophy of leg muscles	50.8	443	46.0	174	49.4	617
Decreased sensation in legs	66.7	657	67.8	320	67.0	977
Decreased reflexes in legs	80.6	780	82.1	329	81.1	1,109
Straight leg raising test	96.9	732	95.3	316	96.4	1,048

*Total for whom status on specified item was known during the reference hospitalization, observed before surgery if any was performed.

tion. Although one cannot assert that the management of military patients was comparable with that of those treated in civilian practice, neurologic consultations generally were done and the clinical evaluation was probably superior. To the extent that definite clinical manifestations of HNP have been documented, it has been shown in Chapter 5 that they affected decisions on choice of therapy to only a limited degree.

In this chapter we will first describe a variety of occupational indices and subjective responses of the physician conducting the follow-up examination, which have different levels of generality in evaluating disability. An attempt will also be made to evaluate disability at the follow-up examination by comparing the specific clinical findings at follow-up for groups of patients exhibiting those findings during the reference hospitalization with the results for groups negative for these findings during that hospitalization. These comparisons will be made separately within treatment groups, not to assess the results of mode of therapy, but to eliminate it as an extraneous variable. The occupational indices and subjective responses will then be used with the clinical signs to obtain a summary index of disability for each patient examined at follow-up. Also described will be an attempt to identify relevant observations during the reference hospitalization that would predict this index and thus be useful in establishing long-term prognosis of lumbar disc patients.

EVALUATION OF INDIVIDUAL VARIABLES

The basic information on clinical signs and symptoms during the reference hospitalization and at the follow-up examination has already been presented in earlier sections (Chapters 3 and 4 and Table 5-6). Of particular interest here are data on the patient's adaptation to his disease, such as the VA disability compensa-

Table 6-2. Percent distribution of patients* by various measures of disability at follow-up and by surgical status during reference hospitalization

Evaluation of disability	HNP surgery at reference hospitalization	No HNP surgery at reference hospitalization	Total
Occupational change from employment history			
Not working now	9.6	6.4	7.7
Change preservice to follow-up	70.5	69.1	69.7
No change preservice to follow-up	19.9	24.5	22.6
Total	100.0	100.0	100.0
Number with known status	322	486	808
Number with unknown status	8	13	21
Occupational change reported by patient as resulting from disc disability			
Change due to disc	50.9	45.9	47.9
No change due to disc	49.1	54.1	52.1
Total	100.0	100.0	100.0
Number with known status	328	492	820
Number with unknown status	2	7	9
Examiner's evaluation of employment handicap			
Handicap	68.3	69.6	69.1
No handicap	31.7	30.4	30.9
Total	100.0	100.0	100.0
Number with known status	325	496	821
Number with unknown status	5	3	8
Examiner's evaluation of use of back			
Limited by weakness	25.8	21.7	23.4
Limited by pain only	45.5	52.3	49.6
Other limitation	4.6	2.2	3.2
Not limited	24.0	23.7	23.8
Total	100.0	99.9	99.9
Number with known status	325	497	822
Number with unknown status	5	2	7
Examiner's evaluation of use of legs			
Limited walking or weight bearing	15.0	16.5	15.9
Cannot run	36.2	39.2	38.0
Other limitation	1.5	1.4	1.5
No limitation	47.2	42.9	44.6
Total	99.9	100.0	100.0
Number with known status	326	497	823
Number with unknown status	4	2	6
Examiner's overall functional impression			
Disability 21 + %	18.5	16.2	17.1
Disability 1% to 20%	61.0	64.7	63.3
No disability from disc	20.5	19.1	19.6
Total	100.0	100.0	100.0
Number with known status	308	482	790
Number with unknown status	22	17	39
VA disability compensation rating at cutoff, June 1961			
Compensated 30 + %†	35.4	19.5	25.1
Compensated 10% to 29%	58.5	60.9	60.1
Claim not filed or disallowed	6.1	19.6	14.8
Total	100.0	100.0	100.0
Number with known status	395	727	1,122
Number with unknown status	0	1	1

*Among 789 patients examined at follow-up and 40 patients with social service interview, except for item on VA disability, compensation rating available for 1,122 men.
†Includes retirement for disability.

Table 6-3. Percent of patients with specified signs at follow-up (FU) examination among those with and without that sign during reference hospitalization by surgical status

| | Surgical status at reference hospitalization | | | |
| | HNP surgery | | No HNP surgery | |
Sign	Same sign present at reference hospitalization	Same sign absent at reference hospitalization	Same sign present at reference hospitalization	Same sign absent at reference hospitalization
Lumbar scoliosis				
Percent positive at FU	17.5	10.5	13.4	14.9
Total number*	126	95	149	134
Significance of difference†	—		—	
Paravertebral muscle spasm				
Percent positive at FU	13.4	11.3	11.5	12.8
Total number	224	71	296	141
Significance of difference	—		—	
Loss of lumbar lordosis				
Percent positive at FU	32.5	27.7	28.2	32.8
Total number	194	101	245	192
Significance of difference	—		—	
Restricted spine motion				
Percent positive at FU	27.5	21.1	28.4	23.7
Total number	149	133	222	190
Significance of difference	—		—	
Weakness of leg muscles				
Percent positive at FU	37.7	37.7	44.8	31.7
Total number	77	106	96	164
Significance of difference	—		$P < .05$	
Atrophy of leg muscles				
Percent positive at FU	62.7	53.1	65.9	62.8
Total number	102	81	123	137
Significance of difference	—		—	
Decreased sensation in legs				
Percent positive at FU	58.4	39.8	55.4	35.3
Total number	178	83	260	136
Significance of difference	$P < .01$		$P < .001$	
Decreased reflexes of knee or ankle				
Percent positive at FU	80.9	61.5	66.4	49.0
Total number	256	52	369	98
Significance of difference	$P < .005$		$P < .005$	

*Percentages are based on these numbers of patients on whom specified sign status could be determined, both from reference hospitalization and from follow-up examination, and who, as indicated in the column headings, either did or did not exhibit the sign at the reference hospitalization.

†P values $\leq .05$ obtained on chi-square tests of significance comparing percent positive between sign status groups; — sign indicates $P > .05$.

tion rating, changes in occupational status, and an overall disability evaluation obtained by the physician conducting the follow-up examination. For these variables Table 6-2 gives comparisons by surgical status. It appears that an appreciable portion of the sample is free of marked disability. Only 7.7% of the patients were unemployed at the time of the follow-up examination, and 52.1% indicated that they did not change employment because of the disc lesion. The examining physicians found no employment handicap in 30.9% and no disability due to disc disease in 19.6%. In the total sample 14.8% of the patients did not file a claim for disability with the VA or had their claim disallowed. For all the above items except VA compensation rating there were no important differences between surgical and nonsurgical patients, but surgical patients did receive high VA compensation ratings more frequently than those with no surgical intervention at the reference hospitalization.

In summary, after more than 20 years, these patients generally experienced only mild to moderate disability. Although they may have changed employment in an effort to adapt to their disease, for the most part they continue to be employed. The 7.7% not working at the time of the examination probably include some individuals between jobs and some unemployed because potential employers would not hire men with a history of treatment for HNP. In the above evaluations of disability, except for the VA compensation rating, no appreciable differences appeared to be associated with surgical status during the reference hospitalization.

It is evident from the data presented here and in previous chapters that disability is considerably less severe at the follow-up examination than during the reference hospitalization, but it is relevant to inquire whether the presence of specific clinical signs during the reference hospitalization affects the frequency with which they will be found at the follow-up examination. The answer is suggested in Table 6-3. There is only a slight tendency for a greater frequency of any given postural sign at follow-up if the sign was present during the reference hospitalization than if it was not present. However, this tendency is not uniform and the differences are not statistically significant. For the neurologic signs there are large and significant differences in the frequencies of decreased sensation in legs, and of decreased reflexes of the knee or ankle, with the presence or absence of these respective signs at the reference hospitalization. Among nonsurgical patients there is a moderate, though barely significant, difference in the frequency of leg weakness at follow-up with the presence or absence of leg weakness at the reference hospitalization.

Particularly remarkable in Table 6-3 are the high frequencies of signs at the follow-up examination among those who did not exhibit them in the first 3 months of the reference hospitalization or before surgery in these 3 months. Except for the two extreme observation points, separated by 20 years, we cannot determine how often these signs have receded or reappeared throughout the follow-up period, although the disease has obviously undergone considerable modification in most patients.

MULTIVARIATE EVALUATION OF DISABILITY AT FOLLOW-UP

At the follow-up examination there were too many measurements of clinical status for a complete evaluation of individual variables against the many observations made during the reference hospitalization. To make such an analysis possible, a principal components analysis of 18 variables from the follow-up examination was performed, and a composite score that measures a general disability factor was computed. The approach used was adapted from published procedures.[1] The disability scores were later used in a multiple regression analysis to predict a patient's disability at follow-up from clinical and other variables observed during the reference hospitalization or at induction into service.

The 18 variables used in the principal components analysis are readily arranged a priori into groups:

A. Examining physician's observations of objective signs and events determined at the time of the follow-up examination
1. Atrophy of muscles of legs
2. Weakness or spasm of muscles of legs
3. Decreased sensation in legs
4. Decreased or absent reflexes of knee or ankle
5. Loss of lumbar lordosis
6. Restriction of motion of lumbar spine
7. Straight leg raising test
8. Changes in occupation from history
B. Examining physician's evaluation of limitation and disability
9. Physician's evaluation of limitation—back pain
10. Physician's evaluation of limitation—back weakness
11. Physician's evaluation of limitation—use of legs
12. Physician's evaluation of degree of handicap in employment
13. Physician's overall functional impression
C. Patient's evaluation of pain and disability
14. Patient's evaluation of back pain
15. Patient's evaluation of leg pain
16. Patient's report of change in employment due to disc
D. Information from VA or private hospital records covering the follow-up period
17. VA compensation rating
18. Surgery for HNP at follow-up

The variables are described in the Appendix. Also specified in the Appendix are the scores used in quantifying each variable and the handling of missing observations (pp. 102 to 105). Data on the examined patients were relatively complete. The occasional missing item of information on an examined patient did not seem to justify the exclusion of all the other data available on him. For each of the variables, scores have therefore been assigned arbitrarily to the missing observations, as indicated in the Appendix. In this manner it was possible to evaluate disability at the follow-up examination for all 789 examined patients.

The means of the 18 variables evaluated at follow-up were compared for patients with and without HNP surgery during the reference hospitalization. In general, differences with operation status are slight. The exceptions are decreased reflexes of knee or ankle, which were more common among the surgical patients; occupational history, which indicated more changes among surgical patients; the

[1]International Business Machines Corporation: System/360 Scientific Subroutine Package, Programmer's Manual, H20-0205-0, White Plains, N. Y., 1966, Technical Publications Department.

Table 6-4. Product moment correlation coefficients for components of disability score for 789 patients with follow-up examination

Variable*	Variable								
	1 Atrophy of legs	2 Weakness of legs	3 Decreased sensation	4 Decreased reflexes	5 Loss of lordosis	6 Restricted motion	7 Straight leg raising test	13 Physician's functional impression	17 VA rating
Clinical signs									
1. Leg atrophy	—							.15	.06
2. Leg weakness	.12	—						.27	.18
3. Decreased sensation	.17	.30	—					.25	.16
4. Decreased reflexes	.08	.12	.23	—				.10	.09
5. Loss of lordosis	.05	.24	.16	.06	—			.26	.15
6. Restricted motion	.07	.11	.10	.08	.17	—		.25	.21
7. SLR test	.05	.22	.13	.09	.12	.29	—	.28	.14
Physician's evaluation									
13. Functional impression								—	.28
9. Limitation—back pain	.16	.17	.23	−.01	.18	.12	.18	.49	.19
10. Limitation—back weak	−.04	.18	.08	.06	.09	−.05	.06	.21	.08
11. Limited use of legs	.16	.27	.26	.17	.19	.24	.31	.50	.25
12. Handicap in employment	.07	.29	.22	.10	.26	.20	.20	.61	.28
Patient's evaluation									
14. Back pain	.04	.16	.13	.00	.16	.17	.18	.31	.14
15. Leg pain	.09	.13	.20	.02	.13	.21	.14	.32	.16
16. Change of employment	.02	.11	.09	.09	.17	.07	.07	.29	.19
Other sources of information									
18. Surgery for HNP at follow-up	.03	.14	.08	.07	.10	.10	.04	.16	.20

*See Appendix for full designation of variables.

VA compensation rating, which was higher for surgical patients; and the patient's complaints of back and leg pains, which were not as extensive among surgical patients.

The 18 variables used in the principal components analysis generally had positive correlations with each other, as measured by product moment coefficients. These coefficients provide a start for the principal components analysis, and their value indicates the degree to which disability on one item is associated with disability on another item. Some of these coefficients are shown in Table 6-4. The three negative correlations are slight and not significant.* A detailed examination of the table indicates that, generally, each variable was correlated most highly with the physician's overall functional impression. Correlations with other judgments of the physician were also appreciable.

The correlation coefficient between the examining physician's functional evaluation and the VA rating of disability is $+.28$, indicating moderate agreement. This is the highest correlation of the VA rating with the other variables. The examining physician's functional evaluation has a higher correlation with all the other variables than does the VA rating of disability, except surgery for HNP at follow-up, which correlates slightly better with the VA rating. It therefore appears that the VA

---

*In addition, the following variables not shown in Table 6-4 have slight negative correlations with changes in occupation determined from the occupational history: muscle atrophy $(-.02)$, decreased sensation $(-.02)$, restriction of motion $(-.01)$, and SLR test $(-.02)$. These correlations are not significantly different from a hypothetical value of zero, indicating an absence of a relationship.

Table 6-5. Correlations of components of disability score with main factor by surgical status for 789 patients with follow-up examination

Variable*	Surgery for HNP at the reference hospitalization	No surgery for HNP at the reference hospitalization	Total
1. Atrophy of legs	.29	.18	.22
2. Weakness of legs	.49	.47	.48
3. Decreased sensation	.37	.48	.44
4. Decreased reflexes	.10	.28†	.21
5. Loss of lordosis	.36	.46	.42
6. Restricted motion	.42	.36	.39
7. SLR test	.50	.40	.42
8. Changes in occupation history	.18	.14	.15
9. Limitation—back pain	.64	.66	.65
10. Limitation—back weakness	.37	.25	.30
11. Limited use of legs	.74	.64†	.68
12. Handicap in employment	.80	.74†	.76
13. Functional evaluation	.79	.74	.76
14. Complaint of back pain	.48	.54	.51
15. Complaint of leg pain	.52	.49	.50
16. Change of employment	.50	.45	.47
17. VA compensation	.58	.37‡	.45
18. Surgery for HNP at follow-up	.28	.17	.21

*See Appendix for full designation of the variables.
†Difference between correlation coefficients of the treatment groups is significant, P <.05.
‡Difference between correlation coefficients of the treatment groups is significant, P <.01.

rating judges disability on the same basis as the physician's functional evaluation, but is not as effective. Both scales use handicap in employment and limitations in the use of the legs as principal criteria of disability. The higher correlations of the physician's functional impression with the other variables can be accounted for in part because the physician himself evaluated disability using the observations that he had made during the physical examination, whereas the VA rating may have been several years old when the observations were made. It is worth noting that the physician's functional evaluation correlates somewhat more highly with the patient's judgments than with any of the clinical variables, whereas the VA rating correlates more highly with weakness of legs (+.18), restriction of back motion (+.21), and surgery for HNP during follow-up (+.20) than with the patient's judgments. However, the scoring of the physician's functional impression appears to produce a more relevant index of disability than that of the VA rating, since the former variable has higher correlations with all the other items except HNP surgery during follow-up.

The purpose of the principal components analysis is to simplify the correlations between variables by identifying independent principal components or factors that best account for the correlations. In this analysis of the 18 variables, five factors were identified and the first has been considered useful in developing a means of quantifying disability.* A factor score (q) was computed for each case by assigning an appropriate weight to each of the 18 variables.† The last column of Table 6-5 shows the correlations of each of the 18 variables with this factor, or factor loadings. The correlations range from +.15 to +.76. It seems that the physician's evaluation of employment handicap is about as useful a measure of disability as the functional impression. Each variable is insufficiently correlated with the factor, for it alone to represent the factor without appreciable loss of information.

Table 6-5 also indicates that when the principal components analysis was done separately for surgical and nonsurgical patients, four variables showed significant differences with surgical status in the factor loadings. The other variables show only small differences in correlations between the two treatment groups. There is some tendency toward higher correlations among patients with surgery during the reference hospitalization, but it is not uniform. The principal components analysis pro-

---

*The first factor in importance accounts for 23.1% of the total variation in the data. The other four, in decreasing order, account for 7.9%, 7.0%, 6.3%, and 5.9%, respectively. All five factors together account for 50.2%. The first factor is therefore considerably more important than any of the factors 2 to 5. The measurement of the latter would probably be subject to considerable sampling error. Since factors 2 to 5 explain only a little of the variation in the measurement of disability, they cannot contribute much to the analysis and they have been disregarded in the subsequent work.

†This score has been computed using the scoring of the individual variables indicated in the Appendix and weighting these scores by coefficients derived from the principal components analysis. If variables are represented by X_1, X_2, . . . X_{18} in the same sequence as given in the Appendix, the equation by which the score is computed is as follows:

$$q = .218X_1 + .489X_2 + .430X_3 + .218X_4 + .447X_5 + .287X_6 + .425X_7 + .142X_8 + .692X_9 + .356X_{10} + .473X_{11} + .640X_{12} + .387X_{13} + .279X_{14} + .250X_{15} + .460X_{16} + .380X_{17} + .276X_{18}$$

The mean value of q is 4.70, the standard deviation is 2.04, and the range is .4 to 9.8.

duced very similar results for surgical and for nonsurgical patients. Therefore, the disability scores based on the experience of the total group are about the same as they would be if scores had been computed separately for surgical and nonsurgical cases, and only the scoring procedure for the total group has been used. The latter score has almost the same mean value for patients with HNP surgery during the reference hospitalization (4.76) as for the nonsurgical patients (4.65). The difference is not significant.

The physician's functional evaluation correlated well with the disability factor (+.76). It therefore seems that the concept of disability from residuals of a herniated nucleus pulposus is valid and that the disability can be measured reasonably well by a single dimension. However, most of the variation in patient disability could not be accounted for by this or any other single factor. Even a five-factor evaluation does not account fully for the disability phenomenon. Apparently, disability from the residuals of HNP is multidimensional, and although it can be assessed with reasonable consistency by a composite index, its full clarification will require further refinement of concepts and observations.

MULTIVARIATE PREDICTION OF DISABILITY

The factor score computed from the factor analysis of follow-up data provides a reasonable index of disability. If variables relevant to prognosis were observed at the earlier stages of the disease or before its manifestation, it should be possible to identify them by examining their relationship to the disability score. Many observations have been obtained before and during the reference hospitalization. So that they would be handled effectively, a multivariate regression analysis was performed. This technique provides a linear combination of the scores of the various independent variables observed before or during the reference hospitalization, which best predicts the dependent variable—the disability score. The prediction is best, in the sense that the sum of squared deviations of the disability score from the value predicted by the regression equation is the smallest possible, using a linear equation. The analysis provides a measure of the relationship of each variable to the disability score. Furthermore, it is possible to evaluate the independent effect of each variable, that is, the effect after variation in the disability score due to other factors has been accounted for.

The regression analysis has been done separately for patients with surgery for HNP during the reference hospitalization and patients treated conservatively. The measures of relationship used are the product moment correlation coefficients. The coefficients showing the relationship of the scores for observations during the reference hospitalization to the scoring of disability at follow-up are shown in Table 6-6.* Among the surgical cases, a significantly (P < .05) greater disability score was noted

---

*The problem of missing information for the variables of interest was more severe during the reference hospitalization than at the follow-up examination. There are no completely satisfactory and generally applicable techniques for the handling of this problem in multivariate analyses. In this work the missing observations were assigned mean values if they were true measurements. If categoric data were scored, the missing observations were assigned the most frequently occurring score or an intermediate score. For several variables the appropriateness of the assigned scores could be questioned. These have been evaluated in separate analyses that are not subject to the restrictive assumptions of the regression analysis.

Table 6-6. Product moment correlation coefficients of observations from reference hospitalization with disability score at follow-up, by surgical status, for 789 patients with follow-up examination

Variable	Surgery for HNP at the reference hospitalization*	No surgery for HNP at the reference hospitalization†	Total‡
Education at entry into service	− .09	− .15	− .12
Age at reference hospitalization	.13	.09	.10
Length of service to reference hospitalization	.12	− .08	− .03
Number of prior relevant admissions	.13	.11	.11
Age at onset of leg pain	.12	.06	.09
Time from leg pain to reference hospitalization	− .01	.06	.03
Duration of reference hospitalization	.14	.02	.08
Extent of leg pain	.01	.02	.02
Back or leg signs prior to reference hospitalization	.01	.11	.07
Loss of lumbar lordosis	.03	.01	.02
Paravertebral muscle spasm	− .03	− .04	− .03
Restriction of motion of lumbar spine	.06	.10	.09
Straight leg raising test	− .01	.03	.02
Muscle weakness of legs	.09	.11	.10
Muscle atrophy of legs	.09	− .03	.02
Decreased sensation in legs	.01	.07	.04
Increased reflexes of knee or ankle	.03	.04	.04
Decreased reflexes of knee or ankle	− .14	.03	− .03
Location of HNP lesion given in final diagnosis	− .06	− .09	− .07
Local osteroarthritis on X-ray before surgery	.04	.02	.03
Myelogram evidence of HNP	− .01	.01	.02
Extent of conservative therapy	.09	− .03	.02
Nature of surgery: fusion	.03	—	—
Nature of surgery: extent of bone removed	.05	—	—
Nature of surgery: multiple interspace	.07	—	—

*Correlations greater than .114 are significant at P <.05, and those greater than .148 are significant at P <.01.
†Correlations greater than .090 are significant at P <.05, and those greater than .118 are significant at P <.01.
‡Correlations greater than .070 are significant at P <.05, and those greater than .092 are significant at P <.01.

with the following reference hospital observations (shown in descending order by strength of relationship):
1. Longer duration of the reference hospitalization
2. "Normal" reflexes of knee and ankle
3. Greater number of previous admissions for conditions related for HNP
4. Greater age at the reference hospitalization
5. Greater length of service to the reference hospitalization
6. Greater age at onset of leg pain

Motor signs, less education, and more intensive conservative therapy are slightly associated with higher disability scores among the surgical patients. There were no significant or appreciable differences in disability at the follow-up examination when analyzed according to the nature of surgical technique; that is, total or partial laminectomy, interlaminar removal, etc., whether single or multiple interspaces were explored, or whether more than one procedure was done.

Among patients treated conservatively, in decreasing order, the strongest statistically significant relationships with greater disability are:

1. Less education
2. Greater number of previous admissions for conditions related to HNP
3. Muscle weakness
4. Indication of clinical findings on back and legs before the reference hospitalization
5. Restriction of back motion
6. Greater age at the reference hospitalization
7. Location of findings at the L4-L5 interspace

Generally, for the same variable, differences in the correlation coefficients of surgical and conservatively treated patients are not significant. Exceptions are as follows: with longer service to the reference hospitalization, there was more disability among surgical patients but less disability among those treated conservatively (P <.01); with decreased reflexes of knee and ankle, there was less disability among surgical patients and very slightly more disability among those treated conservatively (P <.05). However, the relatively large negative correlation in the surgical group suggests that the latter relationship is probably an artifact. A detailed evaluation of various measures of disability did not suggest a convincing explanation of this difference.

Table 6-7 presents the multiple correlation coefficients that measure the proportion of total variation in the disability score explainable by the combined effects of the several variables. On each line the multiple correlation coefficient includes the variable specified for that line and all preceding variables in Table 6-7. Therefore, as one goes from one line down to the next, the value of the multiple correlation

Table 6-7. Multiple and partial correlation coefficients in order in which variables reduced total variance in multiple regression analysis

Variable	Multiple correlation of this and previously entered variables with disability score	Partial correlation with disability score excluding effect of previously entered variables	Significance of partial correlation (P)
	Surgical cases		
Duration of reference hospitalization	.14	+.14	< .05
Decreased reflexes	.20	−.15	< .01
Age at reference hospitalization	.25	+.15	< .01
Muscle weakness	.27	+.11	≃.06
Number of relevant hospitalizations before reference hospitalization	.30	+.12	< .05
	Nonsurgical cases		
Education	.15	−.15	< .01
Muscle weakness	.19	+.12	< .01
Back or leg signs before reference hospitalization	.22	+.11	< .05
Age at reference hospitalization	.24	+.09	< .05
Length of service to reference hospitalization	.26	−.11	< .05
Restriction of motion	.28	+.10	< .05

coefficient increases. The table is arranged so that each new line represents the variable that at that point produces the greatest increase in the multiple regression coefficient. The partial regression coefficients measure the independent effect of each variable, that is, its relationship to the disability score after the effect of the variables previously entered in the table has been excluded from this relationship.

Table 6-7 indicates that when all variables with significant independent predictive value are considered, the disability score can be predicted better than by random guessing, but prediction is still very poor. Among the surgical patients only 9% and among the nonsurgical patients only 8% of the total variation in disability scores can be explained by the variables included in Table 6-7. Nor can the predictive power be increased by including more variables in the regression equations. When ten variables are considered, the proportion of explained variation increases to 12% and 9%, respectively, for the surgical and the nonsurgical patients. But the inclusion of variables without significant partial correlations cannot be justified, since then the model cannot be generalized beyond these specific data.

The most reliable single predictor of future disability among surgical cases is the duration of the reference hospitalization, and among conservatively treated patients, the patient's education. When used singly, however, these variables have little predictive value. Muscle weakness and age during the reference hospitalization contribute to the prediction of disability of both surgical and nonsurgical patients. Among the surgical patients, normal reflexes before surgery and a greater number of prior hospitalizations for conditions related to the back and legs are also independently predictive of increased disability. Among patients treated conservatively, observation of back or leg signs before the reference hospitalization, shorter service to the reference hospitalization, and restriction of back motion independently indicate a significantly worse prognosis.

DISCUSSION

An attempt has been made to evaluate the elements of disability from disc disease and their interrelationships in order to describe the phenomenon more fully and to gain a better understanding of the natural history of lumbar disc disease by identifying factors relevant in long-term prognosis. The picture that emerges from this work appears complex, but a few relationships are definite.

When patients are considered as one group, over a period of 20 years there has been a marked reduction in the overall frequency and intensity of pain and of the postural signs pertaining to the back. Sensory deficits in the legs and decrease or absence of reflexes of knee or ankle occur somewhat less frequently 20 years later than during the original hospitalization, but there is virtually no change in the frequency of atrophy and weakness of leg muscles.

Despite the general trend toward recovery with time, risk of a patient's exhibiting a clinical sign at the follow-up examination is almost as great if this sign was not found at the reference hospitalization as if it was initially present. We hesitate to say in the first instance that the sign originated in the follow-up period and in the second instance that the sign was retained. The observations were made on only two occasions, and the signs may have appeared and subsided repeatedly in the interim. Our observations provide an estimate of the lower limit of this variability, which probably is great. It seems that recovery from lumbar disc disease is a complex process, with configurations of clinical signs arising in the follow-up period with little or no relation to the configuration of signs during the reference hospitalization. The emergence of new clinical signs is not readily explainable, but it must appreciably weaken attempts to predict disability from the signs seen during the reference hospitalization.

At the follow-up examination, considerable disability remains, the disease process appears to continue, and the origin of new signs is not altogether random. The signs noted at the follow-up examination are more strongly associated with each other than those observed during the reference hospitalization. During the reference hospitalization 238 patients had motor, sensory, and reflex signs. The number expected if motor, sensory, and reflex signs occurred independently of each other at that time is 225, which is a slightly and not significantly smaller number than that observed.* There were 249 patients with findings of motor, sensory, and reflex signs at the follow-up examination. Because of the generally lower frequency of the signs at follow-up than at the reference hospitalization, among the 789 patients examined, the number expected if these signs were associated randomly is 186. The latter number is appreciably and significantly smaller (P <.001) than the observed 249 patients with all three types of signs.† The findings reviewed so far indicate that, although the general tendency during the follow-up period was toward recovery, not only did an appreciable number of patients fail to recover, but some became more symptomatic and tended to exhibit all three kinds of neurologic signs. The determining factors in the disease process may have been experiences of the patient during the follow-up period that we were unable to observe in our study.

For some variables, the lack of a strong predictive tendency in the multiple regression analysis could reflect nonlinear relationships in the data or improper assignment of scores. We attempted to detect such conditions by examining the mean disability scores of different groups of particular variables and carrying out an analysis of variance that is not subject to the restrictive assumption of multiple regression analysis. No better predictors of subsequent disability were identified through this analysis that had not appeared in the multiple regression analysis.

It is probably enlightening that, for both patients with and patients without HNP surgery, age at the time of admission had a significant positive relationship

---

*For 549 patients, status with respect to one or more of the signs cannot be determined from the records of the reference hospitalization. This large number with missing observations presents difficulty in establishing the correct expected numbers, since it is apparent that patients free of signs are sometimes classified as having unknown status. The computation used to obtain the expected value of 225 uses information on the 574 patients with known status for all three kinds of signs. An alternative procedure is to determine the total number of patients with motor signs (390), the total with sensory signs (674), and the total with reflex signs (953). Assuming that patients with unknown status for a particular sign are free of that sign allows computation of the expected number with all three kinds of signs as (390/1123) • (674/1123) • (953/1123) • (1123) = 199. This is significantly different (P <.01) from the observed 238. The correct expected number should be between 199 and 225.

†Among the 583 patients whose sign status was determined at follow-up and who *did not* have all three types of neurologic signs during the reference hospitalization, 31.0% had all three types of signs at the follow-up examination. Among the 171 patients examined at follow-up who *did* have all three types of neurologic signs during the reference hospitalization, 39.8% had all three types of signs at follow-up. This difference with neurologic sign status during the reference hospitalization is slight but significant (P <.05).

to subsequent disability and that the relationship is independent of the initial clinical findings. Of the other variables, identified as significant in the two groups, the number of prior hospital admissions for back or leg complaints is equivalent to observations of objective back or leg signs during the earlier service hospitalizations. It seems that the variables that predict long-term disability are largely measures of chronicity of the disease at the time of the reference hospitalization. About one third of the men in the sample had admissions for back or leg complaints, not diagnosed as HNP, antedating the reference hospitalization. In the entire sample, 8.0% of the patients had objective back and leg signs that were noted in the induction physical examination. For 21.0% of the entire group, onset of leg pain occurred before entry into military service. Therefore, it is apparent that many of the cases were not new either at the reference hospitalization or even at induction. In many patients a state was being seen in which the diagnosis had been delayed and in which the evolving syndrome could not be observed directly from the beginning of its natural course. However, it may never be possible to study a large sample without accepting some heterogeneity. We did not succeed in improving the prediction of disability by defining a homogeneous group with onset of disease shortly before the reference hospitalization, possibly because of the small number of patients with recent onset. However, our data suggest important questions about the concepts of this disease and its relationship to other degeneration of the lumbar spine.

SUMMARY

At the follow-up examination, patients generally exhibited only mild to moderate disability. Only 7.7% were unemployed, 69.1% experienced some handicap in their employment, and 85.1% were receiving some amount of disability compensation or pension from the VA. The frequency of postural signs at the follow-up examination was not affected by the presence or absence of these signs at the reference hospitalization. There was some tendency to a higher frequency of neurologic signs at follow-up when these signs were present at the reference hospitalization than when they were absent. Patients for whom follow-up observations were available did not differ in their clinical findings at the reference hospitalization from patients who were not examined or for whom the respective observations were not obtained at the follow-up examination.

Of interest are the relatively high frequencies of specific postural and neurologic signs at the follow-up examination among patients who were free of these signs during the reference hospitalization. It is not possible to predict disability at follow-up usefully from the reference hospital data and other military service information. In separate analyses for patients with and without HNP surgery at the reference hospitalization, the best, though limited, predictors of disability in either group are age at reference hospitalization and indications of leg or back symptoms before the reference hospital admission. The lack of predicability could be due partly to changes in nature of the disease during this long period of follow-up and partly to variation in the stage of the disease at which the reference hospitalizations occurred.

CHAPTER 7

RADIOGRAPHIC DIAGNOSIS

BLAINE S. NASHOLD, JR.

The roentgenographic evaluation of the lumbar spine in this study is unique in that, for some patients, films taken during the Army hospitalization could be compared with films obtained at the follow-up clinical examination 20 years later. Radiographic studies were done during the reference hospitalization on 1,026 of the total sample of 1,123 patients and included myelograms for 604 patients. Interpretations of these films could generally be found in the original records, and they were coded with other data from the reference hospitalization. The films were retired by the Army to the General Services Administration, which determined policy on their disposal. When we attempted to recover the films, it appeared that roentgenograms of the spine for 606 men and myelograms for 379 were still available. The implementation of the film disposal policy cannot be reconstructed at this time. In the evaluation of our data it appears that films are somewhat more often available for men with reference hospital admission in 1945 than for men admitted in 1944, and for men in the intermediate grades than for either privates or commissioned officers. The differences are statistically significant (P <.05) but not large. No significant differences in the availability of radiographic films were noted in relation to the clinical findings during the reference hospitalization, to surgical status, or to participation in the follow-up examination.

The physicians carrying out the follow-up examination were instructed to obtain roentgenograms through the radiology department of their hospitals. Anteroposterior, lateral, and oblique views of the lumbosacral spine were requested. Usable films were obtained on 730 of the 789 patients examined at follow-up. A committee of VA radiologists agreed to review these films and the corresponding roentgenograms from the reference hospitalizations. (The instructions for this review are included in the Appendix, pp. 97 to 101). Among the 760 men with usable follow-up films, 418 (55.0%) had films of the lumbar spine and 271 (35.7%) had myelograms from the reference hospitalization, which were also reviewed. Among the 363 men not included in the radiologic review at follow-up because they were not seen, or if seen did not have usable follow-up films, Army lumbar spine films and myelograms were available for 51.8% and 29.8%, respectively. The differences in the availability of the reference hospital radiologic materials between those included and those not included in the radiologic review are not significant.

A subsample of 75 cases was selected from among the 760 with follow-up roentgenograms reviewed by the radiologists. Cases in the subsample were used in a duplicate review. After they were reviewed and returned by one radiologist, they were included in a shipment of regular cases sent for review to another radiologist. The reviewers were not aware that a duplicate review was being conducted, and there was no way for them to distinguish cases in the subsample from the others. The subsample was selected so that it represented a cross-section of the cases reviewed, with respect to the proportion handled by each reviewer, the time of review, the operative status of the reviewed cases, and the type of radiologic materials available. Included in the duplicate review were service myelograms for 27 men (yielding 54 reviews), service hospital roentgenograms of the lumbar spine for 41 men (yielding 82 reviews), and follow-up roentgenograms for 75 men (yielding 150 reviews). The availability of reference hospital roentgenograms (54.7%) and of myelograms (36.0%) is very similar to that in the total sample of 1,123 patients.

In this chapter we first consider the myelographic evaluation of the disc lesion as carried out during the reference hospitalization and during the review of the myelograms by the VA radiologists, then the evaluation of the follow-up films in relation to the radiologic findings during the reference hospitalization and to the evaluation of disability at follow-up, and finally the results of the duplicate review.

MYELOGRAPHIC EVALUATION

During the reference hospitalization, it was the Army policy that ethyl iodophenylundecylate (Pantopaque) myelography was "for diagnosis as well as for localization of the disc lesion if clinical findings were not adequate for these purposes." The rationale for the test was "to localize the lesion accurately so that removal of the damaged disc could be accomplished with the least possible disturbance of the weight-bearing mechanisms of the spine."[1] In this sample of 1,123

[1]Spurling, R. G.: Management of the ruptured intervertebral disc (herniated nucleus pulposus). In United States Army, Surgery in World War II, vol. II, Neurosurgery, Washington, D. C., 1959, Office of the Surgeon General, Department of the Army.

Table 7-1. Number of patients by status on follow-up review of Army myelogram, by status on reference date,* by status on HNP surgery during reference hospitalization

| Status on follow-up review | Surgical status at reference hospital | | | | | |
| | Surgery for HNP | | No surgery for HNP | | Total | |
	Myelogram before reference date*	Any myelogram at reference hospital	Myelogram before reference date	Any myelogram at reference hospital	Myelogram before reference date	Any myelogram at reference hospital
Myelogram reviewed at follow-up	144	149	110	122	254	271
Myelogram not reviewed at follow-up†	171	180	139	153	310	333
Total with myelogram†	315	329	249	275	564	604
Without myelogram	80	66	479	453	559	519
Total	395	395	728	728	1,123	1,123

*The reference date is the earlier of the date of surgery or the date 3 months after admission to the reference hospital.
†Includes men whose films could not be recovered.

patients, 604 had lumbar myelograms during the reference hospitalization. Of these, 564 were done before the reference date, that is, the earlier of the date of surgery or the date 3 months after admission to the reference hospital. A breakdown by surgical status and status on follow-up review of these films is shown in Table 7-1. More than one myelogram was done for 56 patients. During the follow-up period, 239 myelograms were performed that have not been reviewed in this study.

The Army procedure specified complete removal of the Pantopaque following the examination, although small amounts of contrast medium were noted on the follow-up roentgenograms. Table 7-2 shows the amount of contrast medium, mostly Pantopaque, injected as stated in the reference hospitalization records. Because of the rather broad coding categories, the great majority of cases fall in the 3 to 5 cc. group. According to information in the military medical records, some amount of fluid had been retained in 78.6% of the 420 myelograms for which this information was available. In the review of the follow-up roentgenograms for patients with myelograms at the reference hospitalization, some remaining contrast medium was found in 11.1%, and in 5.2% of the patients with no subsequent myelograms after 1949.

Myelographic films included in the review covered mostly the lower lumbar or midlumbar region (84.5%). Adequate posteroanterior views only were available for 138 patients. For another 118, adequate posteroanterior and oblique views were reviewed. In addition, lateral views were available for 30 patients, all of whom

Table 7-2. Percent of patients by amount of contrast medium injected, determined from service hospital record

Amount injected (cc.)	Percent
< 3	4.1
3 – 5	90.8
6 – 8	4.4
9 +	0.7
Total	100.0
Number with known amount	295*
Number with unknown amount	309
Number with no myelogram	519

*Includes myelograms after reference date. See Table 7-1.

Table 7-3. Location of disc protrusions on Army myelograms reviewed at follow-up

Reviewer's determination of level of lesion	Posterolateral, right	Posterolateral, left	Central
None	146	137	196
L1–L2 only	0	0	1
L2–L3 only	0	1	0
L3–L4 only	5	0	1
L4–L5 only	46	52	30
L5–S1 only	46	59	12
Multiple and other	11	5	3
Total known*	254	254	243

*Excludes myelograms after reference date See Table. 7-1.

also had posteroanterior or oblique views. The level of puncture was at L3-L4 in 66.0%. Needle defects were found for 29.4% of the 252 patients for whom information was available. Of the 261 reviewed films that were given a general interpretation, 5.7% were classified as normal, 22.6% as equivocal, and the remaining 71.6% as abnormal. Partial subdural injections were found in 26 patients, and partial extradural injections in 10 patients. The levels of lesion are given in Table 7-3. It appears that left posterolateral protrusions were most frequent and were evenly divided between the L4-L5 and the L5-S1 levels. About one third of the patients were diagnosed as having central or bilateral lesions. Although 94.3% of the reviewed films were characterized as abnormal, disc protrusions were visualized by the reviewing VA radiologists in only 86.1% of these films.

Table 7-4 summarizes the diagnosis of the level of the HNP lesion as determined from the follow-up review of the Army myelograms, from the myelographic reports in the service record, from clinical observations before surgery, and from operative

Table 7-4. Percent of patients by level of lesion and by source of diagnosis

Level of lesion	Source of diagnosis			
	Follow-up review of Army myelogram*	Army diagnosis of preoperative myelogram*	Clinical diagnosis before myelogram	Surgery for HNP at reference hospitalization
No lesion	13.9	10.3	0.0	0.0
Not L4–S1†	4.5	5.5	5.8	4.6
L4–L5 only	36.9	37.4	31.1	32.9
L5–S1 only	37.3	36.1	46.5	55.9
L4–S1	7.4	10.7	16.6	6.6
Total	100.0	100.0	100.0	100.0
Number with diagnosed level	244	524	241	392
Number with unknown level	10	40	13	3
Total	254	564	254	395

*Before the reference date. See Table 7-1.
†Includes single and multiple levels other than L4-S1 and multiple levels involving L4-L5 or L5-S1, but not both.

Table 7-5. Percent and number of patients by relation of operative findings of HNP to Army myelogram* interpreted during reference hospitalization

Relation of myelogram to operative findings	Percent	Number
Both positive, same level, same side	77.7	240
Both positive, same level, different side	2.6	8
Both positive, different level, same side	8.4	26
Both positive, different level, different side	0.3	1
Both positive, level and side unspecified	5.8	18
Operation positive for HNP, myelogram negative	5.2	16
Total with known status	100.0	309
Total with unknown status	—	6
No myelogram		80
Total	—	395

*Myelograms obtained before the reference date. See Table 7-1.

findings during the reference hospitalization. According to the interpretation of the myelogram by the Army radiologists and in the follow-up review, lesions occurred at the L4-L5 level as often as at the L5-S1 level, When clinical diagnoses and operative findings were considered, more diagnoses were made at the L5-S1 level than at L4-L5. Multiple disc lesions were diagnosed most frequently on the clinical examination and least frequently at surgery.

Surgical and myelographic diagnosis of level of HNP lesion could be compared for 309 of the 395 patients with HNP surgery during the reference hospitalization (Table 7-5). For 74.2% of all surgical patients and for 94.8% of the surgical patients with known myelographic findings, both the Army interpretation of the myelogram and the operative findings were positive. For 77.7% of the myelograms, the findings agreed with the findings on surgery with respect to the level and side of the lesion, and in 80.3% there was agreement on level. Side and level were not specified on the myelogram for 5.8% of the patients, although the myelographic findings were designated as positive. For another 5.2% the myelogram failed to detect any lesion, although one was found surgically.

ROENTGENOGRAPHIC EVALUATION OF LUMBAR SPINE

Included in the follow-up review were 418 Army and 760 follow-up films. The Army films, when available, were sent with the follow-up films to the reviewing radiologist, who probably examined them simultaneously. The results of the review are shown in Table 7-6. Findings of most types of congenital abnormalities in this review were fairly rare; however, spina bifida and asymmetry of articular facets were not uncommon. The frequencies of the various congenital defects were very similar when determined from the Army films and when determined from the follow-up films, but this may reflect in part the simultaneous nature of the review.

Some of the abnormalities classified as acquired in Table 7-6 were noted considerably more often on the follow-up roentgenograms than on the films from the reference hospitalization. No appreciable differences were found in the frequencies of Schmorl's nodes of the vertebral body, limbus vertebra, widened disc space, or fracture of vertebral body between films taken at the two different times. Of particular interest are the high frequencies on the follow-up films of narrow disc space, anterior bony fringing, sclerosis of adjacent surfaces on the body of the vertebra, and kissing spinous process. In addition to the findings presented in Table 7-6 the following numbers of patients were noted with the indicated defects on the Army and on the follow-up films, respectively:

Calcification of disc, central	0, 8
Calcification of disc, posterior	0, 8
Gas in disc (vacuum phenomenon)	1, 78
Posterior bony fringing	4, 150
Neoplasm	2, 6
False joint kissing spinous process	0, 8
Inflammation	1, 3

The greater number of these abnormalities noted on the follow-up films compared with the Army films reflects, in part, the greater number of follow-up films reviewed. However, the observations of gas in the disc and posterior bony fringing are noteworthy.

Analysis-of-variance methods were used to evaluate the relationship of the radiographic findings to disability at the follow-up examination. During the refer-

Table 7-6. Percent of patients with positive findings as determined in radiologic review at follow-up by type of finding and time of film

Type of finding	Percent positive on Army films	Percent positive on follow-up films
Congenital abnormalities		
Spina bifida	11.5	10.7
Spondylolysis	4.5	6.4
Spondylolisthesis—any severity	0.5	1.5
Transitional vertebra { Sacralization, L5	3.3	5.0
{ Lumbarization, S1	6.0	6.4
Congenital flat pedicles, right	6.0	6.4
Congenital flat pedicles, left	5.5	6.2
Asymmetry of articular facets, L5–S1 only	19.9	20.8
Other than above	2.6	2.6
Acquired abnormalities		
Schmorl's nodes of vertebral body	7.2	8.8
Limbus vertebra	5.0	4.6
Unusually wide disc space	3.3	4.6
Unusually narrow disc space	30.6	68.4
Narrow lumbosacral space	9.8	23.2
Bony fringing—anterior	7.4	56.3
Sclerosis of adjacent surfaces of vertebral body	1.7	23.6
Lumbar arthritis		
Of articular facets, right	1.4	19.1
Of articular facets, left	2.2	19.2
Rheumatoid arthritis or ankylosing spondylitis	0.0	0.7
Kissing spinous process, simple	2.4	14.9
Arthritic changes of sacroiliac joint	5.0	10.4
Vertebral fracture, body	1.0	1.8
Total number reviewed	418	760

ence hospitalization the only radiographic abnormalities sufficiently prevalent for analysis with the disability scoring described in Chapter 4 were asymmetry of articular facets and unusual narrowing of the disc space. No significant increase in disability at follow-up was evident with the asymmetry of articular facets on the Army films. The mean disability score was 5.04 ± .20 for patients on whose Army roentgenograms unusual narrowing of the disc space was noted, whereas the mean was 4.54 ± .12 among patients with no unusual narrowing. The difference, though significant (P < .05), is not large. On the follow-up roentgenograms a significantly higher mean disability score was obtained for patients who had findings of anterior bony fringing (4.94 ± .10), compared to those without this finding (4.47 ± .11). This is also a modest difference but P < 0.001. No differences in the mean disability score were noted with the presence or absence on the follow-up roentgenograms of asymmetry of articular facets, narrowing of the disc space, sclerosis of adjacent surfaces of the vertebral body, arthritis of articular facets, and kissing spinous process.

DUPLICATE REVIEW

The subsample used in the duplicate review consisted of myelograms for 27 men, reference hospital roentgenograms for 41, and follow-up films for 75. The

Table 7-7. Number of positive findings in duplicate review of reference hospital and of follow-up roentgenograms and number positive on agreeing reviews by nature of finding

Nature of finding	Reference hospital roentgenograms		Follow-up roentgenograms	
	Number positive*	Number of agreements on positive†	Number positive*	Number of agreements on positive†
Congenital abnormalities				
Spina bifida	12	6	19	10
Spondylolysis	3	0	9	0
Transitional vertebra	13	8	21	8
Congenital flat pedicles, right	8	0	12	0
Congenital flat pedicles, left	8	2	12	2
Acquired abnormalities				
Schmorl's nodes of vertebral body	6	2	12	0
Limbus vertebra	4	2	6	2
Unusually wide disc space	3	0	6	0
Unusually narrow disc space	26	6	97	62
Narrow lumbosacral space	10	2	32	10
Bony fringing—anterior	5	2	74	50
Sclerosis of adjacent surfaces of vertebral body	0	–	28	10
Lumbar arthritis				
Of articular facets, right	1	0	25	2
Of articular facets, left	1	0	27	2
Rheumatoid arthritis or ankylosing spondylitis	0	–	0	—
Kissing spinous process, simple	3	0	22	2

*Counted are positive findings on individual reviews for films evaluated by pairs of reviewers.
†Counted are positive findings by a pair of reviewers; each agreement contributes a count of two.

reviewers classified as abnormal all myelogram films included in the subsample except one. Therefore, there was no possibility of a greater disagreement on the general interpretation. For most items the frequency of specific findings in the 54 myelogram reviews was low, and when any was reported by one radiologist, there was seldom confirmation by the other. The total number of abnormalities noted by either reviewer, and the number agreed on by both members of the reviewing pairs, are given, respectively, below*:

Congenitally narrow space	3, 0
Ligamentum flavum defect	5, 2
Central disc protrusions	8, 4
Swollen nerve roots	3, 0
Posterolateral protrusions, right	16, 12
Posterolateral protrusions, left	19, 14

Information on the results of the duplicate review of the Army and VA films is given in Table 7-7. The frequencies of positive findings in the review of all materials compare well with the frequencies of positive findings in the duplicate review. The films taken during the reference hospitalization were generally judged to show

*The agreements are counted as two observations of the abnormality.

few positive findings, and the frequency of confirmation of these positive findings is low. At the follow-up examination, the frequency of positive findings is higher for most items than on the earlier roentgenograms. For some items the frequency of abnormalities at follow-up is sufficiently high to affect the interpretation of the number of findings confirmed. For example, abnormal narrowing of the disc space was found in 97 of the 150 reviews. With this frequency of positive findings, we would expect 62 agreements (31 pairs of reviews), the number actually observed in Table 7-7, to agree on the basis of chance alone.* It probably is not quite correct to represent the radiologic review by a model in which the reviewers randomly distribute 97 positive findings. But the frequencies of confirmation are sufficiently low that radiologic information can have only limited usefulness in prognostic and clinical evaluations.

DISCUSSION

The roentgenograms showed definite degenerative changes of the lumbosacral spine after 20 years, which confirms that the syndrome of the herniated lumbosacral disc is often associated with such degenerative changes. The origin of these changes, how they become initiated, and how they progress are not understood.

The occurrence of HNP in male members of the same family seems to point to a possible hereditary or congenital association. There are no clinical or radiographic studies that show a sex-linked difference in the incidence of congenital spinal abnormalities of the lumbosacral region. HNP has been noted to occur with greater frequency in males, but this has usually been explained by the greater risk of back trauma among males because of the nature of their employment. In his extensive study of herniated disc disease, Hanraets[2] comments that it is not a given anomaly that is heritable but a tendency of the spinal column to develop anomalies. The congenital vertebral anomalies—such as spina bifida, spondylosis, and transitional vertebra—occurred in the veterans studied in our series at about the same frequency as reported in the literature.[3,4] The congenital bony defects noted on roentgenograms do not appear to be associated with the presence of HNP in our group. The following roentgenographic signs commonly appear in association with lumbosacral disc degeneration: narrowing of the intervertebral disc space, reactive changes in the region of the joints at the involved spinal level, the vacuum phenomenon, calcification in the intervertebral disc space, vertebral instability, posterior displacement of vertebra (pseudospondylolisthesis), abnormal mobility of vertebrae, and changes in the lumbar axis. The present study showed a significant increase on the follow-up films in the frequency of narrowing of the lumbosacral disc space, vacuum phenomenon, bony fringing and sclerosis of the vertebral bodies, and changes in the articular facets. Despite the increased frequency of these roentgenographic signs, no hint exists as to their etiology.

---

*75 • $(97/150)^2 = 31.4$.

[2]Hanraets, P. R. M. J.: The degenerative back and its differential diagnosis, Amsterdam, 1959, Elsevier Publishing Co.

[3]Friedman, M. M., Fischer, F. J., and Van Demark, R. E.: Lumbosacral roentgenograms of one hundred soldiers. A control study, Amer. J. Roentgen. **55**:292-298, 1946.

[4]Crow, N. E., and Brogdon, B. G.: The "normal" lumbosacral spine, Radiology **72**:97, 1959.

Williams and Fullenlove[5] made a roentgenographic comparison between 200 laborers without back symptoms and 68 persons with proved HNP at operation. They listed the rate for narrowing of the disc space, flatness of the lordotic curve, scoliosis, and localized hypertrophic spurs found in the two groups. They noted that narrowing of the disc space and spur formation seemed to be the two most prominent roentgenographic findings associated with lumbar disc lesions. Similar findings were noted in the present study, with a more than twofold increase in the frequency of narrowed disc space and a sevenfold increase in the frequency of bony fringing or spur formation during the period of follow-up. Butler,[6] in an evaluation of 200 unselected persons with acute or chronic low back pain, noted that 26% had evidence of hypertrophic arthritis; 9%, Marie-Strumpell arthritis; 13%, spina bifida; and 15%, facet abnormalities.

The influence of erect posture, with its stresses and strains centered on the lumbosacral spine, has been considered as one cause of degeneration of the lumbar discs. It has been hypothesized that the change of man's mode of locomotion as he developed from an arboreal animal to an erect terrestial biped has weakened the lumbosacral spine. Combined with the change in posture, repeated small traumatic insults increase the susceptibility of the spine and discs to degeneration. The only experimental work to support this idea is that of Yamada,[7,8] who carried out an experimental study of intervertebral disc herniation in bipedal rats and mice. The bipedal animal changes its mode of locomotion from the quadriped stance to walking on its hind legs. He noted the development of degenerated lumbar discs in the bipedal animals within 12 to 24 months, but no degeneration in the control group. He also showed that there were great mechanical stresses on the sacroiliac portion of the spinal column in the bipedal animals that he believed resulted in intervertebral disc herniation. This interesting experimental evidence supports the idea that man's erect posture predisposes him to disc degeneration.

The use of contrast Pantopaque myelography in the diagnosis of HNP has been common since its introduction in 1940. The procedure over the years has proved safe. Although the removal of contrast media at the end of the examination is important, small amounts of dye are generally retained. It has been stated that the dye is usually absorbed in several years. In this study, in more than 5% of the patients, the dye was noted in the spinal canal 12 to 20 years after the last myelogram; however, there was no evidence of adverse effects of retention of these small amounts of contrast medium. The myelograms were carried out routinely in the Army to localize lesions accurately, so that surgery could be confined to the level of a damaged disc. Our data bear out the reliability of myelograms in relation to surgical diagnosis. These findings are comparable with those of other studies. Persons with well-defined symptoms and clinical findings can be operated on without myelography, but where any doubt exists, myelography is important. The ac-

[5]Williams, A. J., and Fullenlove, T.: Herniation of intervertebral discs; an evaluation of the indirect signs, Calif. Med. **83:**433-434, 1955.
[6]Butler, E.: Low back pain and its management by the general surgeons, Calif. Med. **68:**70-74, 1948.
[7]Yamada, K.: The dynamics of experimental posture. Experimental study of intervertebral disc herniation in bipedal animals, Clin. Orthop. **25:**20-31, 1962.
[8]Yamada, K.: The dynamics of experimental posture. Experimental study of intervertebral disc herniation in bipedal animals, Tokushima J. Exp. Med. **8:**350-361, 1962.

curacy of myelography diminishes in patients with previous laminectomy, in whom it may be misleading. If the lumbar spinal canal is unusually widened, the herniation of the disc will often be missed, so that evaluation of the clinical signs and symptoms becomes important.

The small duplicate review of radiographic materials revealed a remarkably low level of agreement between the reviewing radiologists on most of the items indicating lumbar spine degeneration. Unfortunately, it was not possible to carry out a comparable replication of the follow-up clinical examination. The lack of strong prognostic indicators in lumbar disc disease may be due in part to the limited reliability of the observations both originally and at follow-up. However, despite the demonstrated unreliability of the radiologic evaluation, it is clearer from the radiologic data than from the clinical observations that over the 20-year follow-up period many of the patients experienced degenerative diseases of the lumbar spine other than disc herniation. It remains for another study to determine the extent to which the degenerative changes are a reflection of normal aging and the extent to which they are related specifically to disc herniation.

SUMMARY

In this study 418 roentgenograms taken during the reference hospitalization were available for comparison with roentgenograms made at the clinical examination 20 years later. Myelograms were routinely done before surgery during the reference hospitalization, and 271 of them were evaluated as part of the follow-up review. Some residual Pantopaque was visible in 5% of the films obtained 20 years after the myelogram. However, there was no clinical evidence that the retained dye had been accompanied by complications. In 80% of the patients the findings at operation ageed with the myelographic defect, and in only 5% did the myelogram fail to detect a lesion that was found later at surgery.

The number of congenital defects of the lumbar spine in this group of men corresponds closely with that reported in other radiographic studies of patients with HNP. Of interest was an increase in spinal degenerative changes noted in the lumbosacral region after a period of 20 years. The most common findings were narrowed disc space, Schmorl's nodes, limbus vertebra, and arthritic changes in the facets of the lumbosacral spine. Unfortunately, radiographic studies of the lumbar spine have not been commonly reported in the general literature, so that comparisons could not be made with other groups of HNP patients or with groups not selected for degenerative diseases of the spine.

CHAPTER *8*

FINAL SUMMARY

BLAINE S. NASHOLD, JR., and ZDENEK HRUBEC

The study presented here consists of a 20-year clinical follow-up of Army personnel initially hospitalized with a first service diagnosis of herniated lumbar disc during 1944-1945. We have analyzed the history, the neurologic and orthopedic clinical findings, and the roentgenographic evaluations of films from both the service hospitalization and the subsequent follow-up examination. A definitive model of the natural history of lumbar disc disease did not emerge from this work; indeed it appears that the disease is more complex than had been generally thought. Certain symptoms and signs were noted consistently, and their patterns seem to represent a degree of uniformity in the clinical expression of the disc syndrome. Fluctuations in the progress of lumbar disc disease are known to occur over time, but the full extent of such fluctuations could be even greater than we observed in these patients because our data cover only two brief time periods, separated by about 20 years.

From an evaluation of the family histories it does seem that lumbar disc disease occurs predominantly in male family members, which may reflect a higher prevalence among males than among females. The patients' own histories reveal a collateral occurrence of thoracic and cervical disc herniation and perhaps of disorders of connective tissue such as bursitis and hypertrophic arthritis. These findings confirm what clinicians treating disc disease have long suspected. In the present study, lumbar disc disease initially appeared as a cluster of characteristic symptoms that included pain, usually first localized to the lower back and later referred to one or the other leg. At the time of hospital admission, back pain and leg pain were almost always both present. There was a predominance of leg pain on the left, but the reason for this is not clear. Physical stresses that tended to focus on the lower spine and its mobility, such as lifting or jumping, seemed to precipitate the initial clinical signs and symptoms, and physical activity often set off the chain of events leading to the reference hospitalization. When the pain radiated into the leg, the sciatic nerve usually was tender to palpation. Associated with the leg pain was restriction of spinal motion, generally toward the side of the leg pain. After 20 years the leg pain had generally subsided, and in an appreciable proportion of the patients it had disappeared completely; but back pain, although decreased in severity, continued to persist in most persons.

The clinical signs of HNP can be divided into neurologic and postural. The frequency of both types was high at the initial hospitalization, but the frequency of postural signs diminished markedly with time. The postural findings included scoliosis, tilt of the spine, muscle spasm, loss of lumbar lordosis, and restriction of lumbar spinal motion. Muscle spasm and restriction of spinal motion were particularly frequent. Generally they occurred together at the initial hospitalization, and when one was noted the other was more likely to be present. Although the postural symptoms did diminish significantly over the 20-year period, the patients were likely to retain some neurologic signs. The frequency of atrophy and weakness of leg muscle was high initially, and at the follow-up examination motor signs were particularly common, which suggests that motor nerves are lastingly affected by disc compression. Diminished sensation could be detected at the follow-up examination in about half of the patients, but weakness of leg muscles gave a somewhat better index of the patient's physical disability at follow-up, and when seen at the reference hospitalization muscle weakness was significantly though slightly related to prognosis. The reflex signs and sensory changes are not very accurate means of localizing the level of the lesion, either initially or 20 years later. In addition to those already mentioned, signs such as positive straight leg raising, or positive crossed straight leg raising, occurred in a high percentage of these patients at the reference hospitalization. Of interest is the fairly frequent occurrence of signs at the follow-up examination among patients free of those signs initially. This finding suggests the presence of a continuing pathologic or adaptive process that can be evaluated fully only with regular periodic reexamination.

The clinical signs can persist for long periods of time even after the initial back and sciatic pain has subsided or disappeared. However, examination of a patient 20 years later did not give the examining physician much basis for judging the initial severity of the disease, nor was it possible to identify variables at the reference hospitalization that were especially useful in prognosis. Judgment of the degree of disability is best made on the basis of handicap in employment, overall clinical impression of the patient's functional disability, subjective symptoms, and motor signs. The current methods employed in rating the disability of patients with lumbar disc disease need reevaluation.

The comparative value of surgical versus conservative management could not be dealt with directly in this study. The technique of surgery in disc disease has been evolving over the past 20 years. Army surgeons were conservative in their surgical removal of the disc fragment, surgery was sometimes undertaken only after prolonged attempts at conservative treatment, and the patients who were operated on tended to be more affected by the disease than the patients treated conservatively. Conservative therapy then, as now, was not well defined. In the absence of a rigorous therapeutic control, with randomization of patients to different treatment modes, one could not hope for a critical comparison of surgical versus conservative treatment. Certainly pain was immediately relieved in a significant percentage of the patients by operation, and the complaint of pain continues to be of major importance when surgical exploration is under consideration. Spinal lumbar fusion, which has become an adjunct in the treatment of chronic lumbar disc disease, cannot be assessed because of the small number of fusions in this group. Patients with initial intractable sciatica plus motor symptoms appear to be best treated surgically, but surgery may not relieve motor signs; these may persist for a long time and play a role, although a limited one, in the development of disability.

Radiographic films of the lumbar spine and myelograms provide important information for the clinical evaluation of patients with lumbar disc disease. In this study, changes in the spine, seen over a 20-year period, provide dramatic evidence of degeneration of the joints, ligaments, and disc spaces in the lumbar region. The exact relevance of these findings to the natural history of the disease is not clear, as there are no comparative radiologic studies in normal subjects. It would seem important to carry out long-range radiographic studies on normal persons, as well as on those with varying kinds of spinal pathology, so that nonspecific aging effects could be distinguished from processes specific to the various diseases affecting the spine. Radiographic interpretation of spinal films seemed to consist of somewhat arbitrary judgments by the radiologist, based on his past experience. There is a need for more objective means of analyzing roentgenographic spinal pathology. A methodologic strengthening of roentgenographic observations of this nature could be of prime importance in future studies, possibly giving insight into the etiologic and historical mechanisms of lumbar disc disease.

The usefulness of the lumbar myelogram as a diagnostic tool was confirmed in these patients even though in 1944-1945 the myelogram had only recently been introduced into clinical practice. Myelography is a safe procedure with few side effects as judged in these men 20 years later. The dye may not be absorbed as quickly or completely as has been previously suggested. In a small percentage of subjects the dye was visible on the roentgenograph after long periods of time, which emphasizes the importance of its complete removal at the time of the myelogram.

The current study raises more questions than it answers and this is not unexpected. Lumbar disc disease may not be a single clinical entity, nor need one causal factor such as heredity, or degenerative or functional change, be responsible for the occurrence of the disease in every person. The answers to these questions could be arrived at in the future, and we hope that this study will serve as a guidepost for subsequent investigations.

APPENDIX

ABSTRACTING OF RECORDS OF THE REFERENCE HOSPITALIZATION, OF OTHER MILITARY RECORDS, AND OF VA RECORDS

For all men eligible for the study, the staff of the Follow-up Agency (FUA) reviewed the service personnel and medical records and records of VA claims and hospitalizations. Nonmedical data from military service records and results of the induction physical examination were recorded on form FUA R20-1. The accompanying "Abstracting work sheet" (FUA R20-11) was filled out for each man, showing a brief history of symptoms and factors related to onset of lumbar disc disease. Also recorded were findings on the neurologic examination during the reference hospitalization and a history of any disability pension or compensation rating by the VA. The information from the work sheet was then put in coded form onto the accompanying forms FUA R20-7 and FUA R20-8. Reports on roentgenograms or on myelographic studies were reviewed and coded directly onto form FUA R20-7. Information on subsequent hospitalizations for back or leg symptoms related to HNP was coded directly onto the accompanying form FUA R20-9. Pertinent portions of the medical records were copied for later review by the participating physicians. These included history of the illness, complete neurologic examinations, radiographic and myelographic reports, reports of surgery, and the final summary from the reference hospitalization.

NAS-NRC
FUA R20-1
July 1960

NATURAL HISTORY OF LUMBAR DISC LESIONS

Information From Military Service Records

Roster _____

Case No. _____

I. Identification	SN	VA No.
Name		

II. Dates — Day Month Year — III. Preservice history

	Day	Month	Year			
A. Date of birth				A. Place of birth _____		C. Urban-rural
B. EAD WW II				B. Residence at EAD Postal address (Box No., or RFD)_____ City or county and State _____		D. Marital status
C. Reference point						
D. Arrival O/S						E. Race
E. Separation						

F. Education (years completed)
Elementary_____
High school_____
College _____ _____

G. Employment
1. Occupation_____
3. Duties performed _____
2. Years in this occupation_____
4. Average earnings $_____ per_____
5. Business of employer_____

IV. EAD physical examination

A. Height_____inches
B. Weight_____pounds

C. Girths
  1. Nipples Inspiration____inches
  2. Nipples Expiration____inches
  3. Umbilicus ____inches

D. Posture
Good_____
Fair_____
Poor_____

E. Frame
Heavy_____
Medium_____
Light_____
Other_____

F. Defects at EAD

V. Information from service record—military history

A. Blood type	C. MOS changes prior to reference point			D. Rank changes prior to RP	
	Specialty—name	Number	Date assigned	Rank	Date assigned
B. Religion					

E. Organizations prior to RP to which assigned or attached, Z/I and O/S (including Service Schools)				F. Campaigns (combat credit)	G. Sports and hobbies
	Day	Month	Year		
				VI. Separation reason or CDD diagnosis	

R-20	**LUMBAR DISC LESIONS—ABSTRACTING WORK SHEET**	NAS-NRC FUA R20-11 May 1961

Case No._____

Name_____

Examinations (N = Normal)

History of injuries and pain			
	Scoliosis		
	Tilt or list		
	Restricted: Flexion		
	Extension		
	Rotation		
	Lat. bend.		
	Loc. percussion		
	Jug. compression		
	Lordosis		
	Loc. tenderness		
	Paravertebral muscle spasm		
	SLR: Right		
	Left		
	Lasègue: Right		
	Left		
	Sensation		
VA rating			
	Sciatic tenderness		
	Muscle strength		
	Muscle atrophy		
	Thigh meas.		
	Calf meas.		
	AJ: Right		
	Left		
	KJ: Right		
	Left		
	Other		

Form FUA R20–7

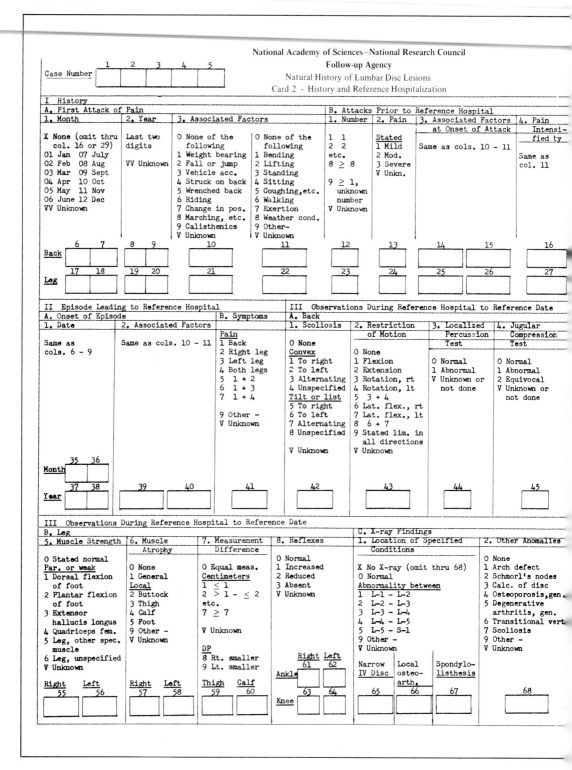

National Academy of Sciences–National Research Council
Follow-up Agency
Natural History of Lumbar Disc Lesions
Card 2 - History and Reference Hospitalization

Case Number 1 2 3 4 5

I History

A. First Attack of Pain

1. Month

X None (omit thru col. 16 or 29)
01 Jan
02 Feb
03 Mar
04 Apr
05 May
06 June
VV Unknown

07 July
08 Aug
09 Sept
10 Oct
11 Nov
12 Dec

2. Year

Last two digits

VV Unknown

3. Associated Factors

0 None of the following
1 Weight bearing
2 Fall or jump
3 Vehicle acc.
4 Struck on back
5 Wrenched back
6 Riding
7 Change in pos.
8 Marching, etc.
9 Calisthenics
V Unknown

0 None of the following
1 Bending
2 Lifting
3 Standing
4 Sitting
5 Coughing, etc.
6 Walking
7 Exertion
8 Weather cond.
9 Other–
V Unknown

B. Attacks Prior to Reference Hospital

1. Number

1 1
2 2
etc.
8 ≥ 8
9 ≥ 1, unknown number
V Unknown

2. Pain

Stated
1 Mild
2 Mod.
3 Severe
V Unkn.

3. Associated Factors at Onset of Attack

Same as cols. 10 - 11

4. Pain Intensified by

Same as col. 11

Back: 6 7 | 8 9 | 10 | 11 | 12 | 13 | 14 | 15 | 16

Leg: 17 18 | 19 20 | 21 | 22 | 23 | 24 | 25 | 26 | 27

II Episode Leading to Reference Hospital

A. Onset of Episode

1. Date

Same as cols. 6 - 9

Month: 35 36

Year: 37 38

2. Associated Factors

Same as cols. 10 - 11

39 40

B. Symptoms

Pain
1 Back
2 Right leg
3 Left leg
4 Both legs
5 1 + 2
6 1 + 3
7 1 + 4

9 Other –
V Unknown

41

III Observations During Reference Hospital to Reference Date

A. Back

1. Scoliosis

0 None
Convex
1 To right
2 To left
3 Alternating
4 Unspecified
Tilt or list
5 To right
6 To left
7 Alternating
8 Unspecified
V Unknown

42

2. Restriction of Motion

0 None
1 Flexion
2 Extension
3 Rotation, rt
4 Rotation, lt
5 3 + 4
6 Lat. flex., rt
7 Lat. flex., lt
8 6 + 7
9 Stated lim. in all directions
V Unknown

43

3. Localized Percussion Test

0 Normal
1 Abnormal
V Unknown or not done

44

4. Jugular Compression Test

0 Normal
1 Abnormal
2 Equivocal
V Unknown or not done

45

III Observations During Reference Hospital to Reference Date

B. Leg

5. Muscle Strength

0 Stated normal
Par. or weak
1 Dorsal flexion of foot
2 Plantar flexion of foot
3 Extensor hallucis longus
4 Quadriceps fem.
5 Leg, other spec. muscle
6 Leg, unspecified
V Unknown

Right 55 Left 56

6. Muscle Atrophy

0 None
1 General
Local
2 Buttock
3 Thigh
4 Calf
5 Foot
9 Other –
V Unknown

Right 57 Left 58

7. Measurement Difference

0 Equal meas.
Centimeters
1 ≤ 1
2 > 1 - ≤ 2
etc.
7 ≥ 7

V Unknown

DP
8 Rt. smaller
9 Lt. smaller

Thigh 59 Calf 60

8. Reflexes

0 Normal
1 Increased
2 Reduced
3 Absent
V Unknown

Right 61 Left 62
Ankle

Right 63 Left 64
Knee

C. X-ray Findings

1. Location of Specified Conditions

X No X-ray (omit thru 68)
0 Normal
Abnormality between
1 L-1 - L-2
2 L-2 - L-3
3 L-3 - L-4
4 L-4 - L-5
5 L-5 - S-1
9 Other –
V Unknown

Narrow IV Disc 65 | Local osteo-arth. 66 | Spondylo-listhesis 67

2. Other Anomalies

0 None
1 Arch defect
2 Schmorl's nodes
3 Calc. of disc
4 Osteoporosis, gen.
5 Degenerative arthritis, gen.
6 Transitional vert.
7 Scoliosis
9 Other –
V Unknown

68

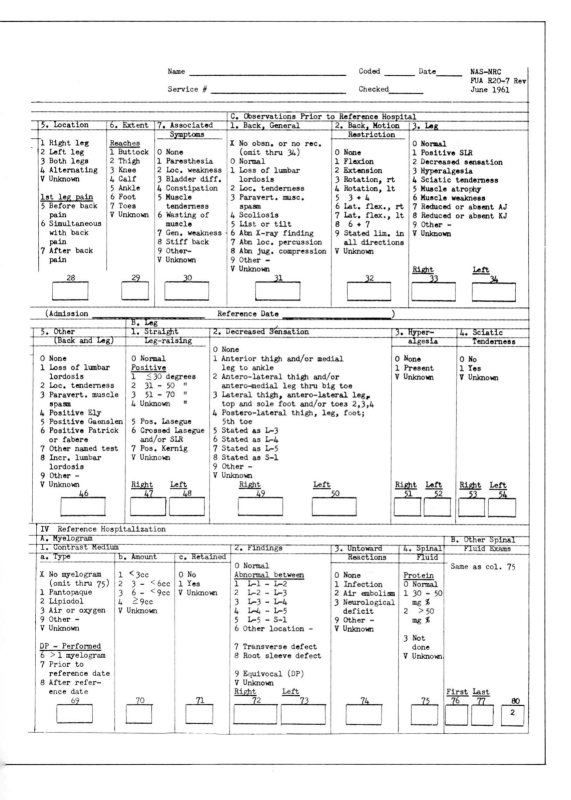

Name _____   Coded _____ Date_____   NAS—NRC
                                                                       FUA R20-7 Rev
      Service # _____   Checked_____   June 1961

C. Observations Prior to Reference Hospital

5. Location	6. Extent	7. Associated Symptoms	1. Back, General	2. Back, Motion Restriction	3. Leg
1 Right leg 2 Left leg 3 Both legs 4 Alternating V Unknown 1st leg pain 5 Before back pain 6 Simultaneous with back pain 7 After back pain 28	Reaches 1 Buttock 2 Thigh 3 Knee 4 Calf 5 Ankle 6 Foot 7 Toes V Unknown 29	0 None 1 Paresthesia 2 Loc. weakness 3 Bladder diff. 4 Constipation 5 Muscle tenderness 6 Wasting of muscle 7 Gen. weakness 8 Stiff back 9 Other- V Unknown 30	X No obsn. or no rec. (omit thru 34) 0 Normal 1 Loss of lumbar lordosis 2 Loc. tenderness 3 Paravert. musc. spasm 4 Scoliosis 5 List or tilt 6 Abn X-ray finding 7 Abn loc. percussion 8 Abn jug. compression 9 Other - V Unknown 31	0 None 1 Flexion 2 Extension 3 Rotation, rt 4 Rotation, lt 5 3 + 4 6 Lat. flex., rt 7 Lat. flex., lt 8 6 + 7 9 Stated lim. in all directions V Unknown 32	0 Normal 1 Positive SLR 2 Decreased sensation 3 Hyperalgesia 4 Sciatic tenderness 5 Muscle atrophy 6 Muscle weakness 7 Reduced or absent AJ 8 Reduced or absent KJ 9 Other - V Unknown Right Left 33 34

(Admission _____   Reference Date _____)

B. Leg

5. Other (Back and Leg)	1. Straight Leg-raising	2. Decreased Sensation	3. Hyper-algesia	4. Sciatic Tenderness
0 None 1 Loss of lumbar lordosis 2 Loc. tenderness 3 Paravert. muscle spasm 4 Positive Ely 5 Positive Gaenslen 6 Positive Patrick or fabere 7 Other named test 8 Incr. lumbar lordosis 9 Other - V Unknown 46	0 Normal Positive 1 ≤30 degrees 2 31 - 50 " 3 51 - 70 " 4 Unknown " 5 Pos. Lasegue 6 Crossed Lasegue and/or SLR 7 Pos. Kernig V Unknown Right Left 47 48	0 None 1 Anterior thigh and/or medial leg to ankle 2 Antero-lateral thigh and/or antero-medial leg thru big toe 3 Lateral thigh, antero-lateral leg, top and sole foot and/or toes 2,3,4 4 Postero-lateral thigh, leg, foot; 5th toe 5 Stated as L-3 6 Stated as L-4 7 Stated as L-5 8 Stated as S-1 9 Other - V Unknown Right Left 49 50	0 None 1 Present V Unknown Right Left 51 52	0 No 1 Yes V Unknown Right Left 53 54

IV Reference Hospitalization

A. Myelogram

1. Contrast Medium			2. Findings	3. Untoward Reactions	4. Spinal Fluid	B. Other Spinal Fluid Exams
a. Type	b. Amount	c. Retained				
X No myelogram (omit thru 75) 1 Pantopaque 2 Lipiodol 3 Air or oxygen 9 Other - V Unknown DP - Performed 6 >1 myelogram 7 Prior to reference date 8 After reference date 69	1 <3cc 2 3 - <6cc 3 6 - <9cc 4 ≥9cc V Unknown 70	0 No 1 Yes V Unknown 71	0 Normal Abnormal between 1 L-1 - L-2 2 L-2 - L-3 3 L-3 - L-4 4 L-4 - L-5 5 L-5 - S-1 6 Other location - 7 Transverse defect 8 Root sleeve defect 9 Equivocal (DP) V Unknown Right Left 72 73	0 None 1 Infection 2 Air embolism 3 Neurological deficit 9 Other - V Unknown 74	Protein 0 Normal 1 30 - 50 mg % 2 >50 mg % 3 Not done V Unknown 75	Same as col. 75 First Last 76 77 80 2

Form FUA R20–8

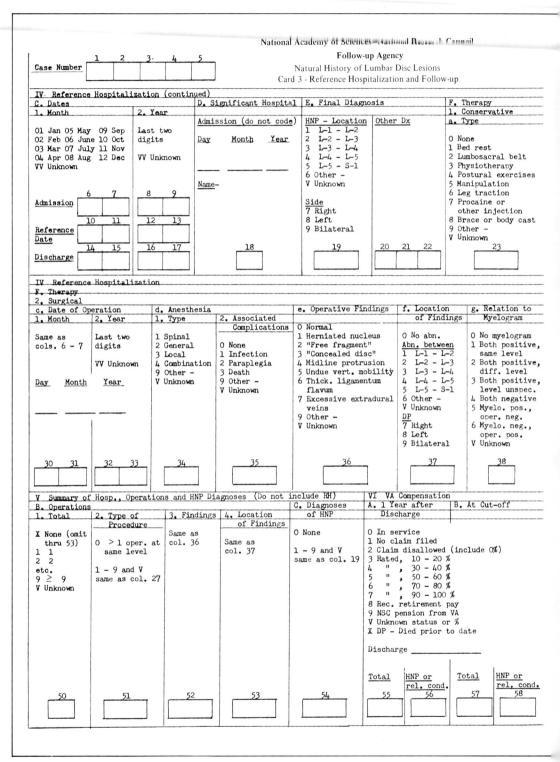

National Academy of Sciences—National Research Council
Follow-up Agency
Natural History of Lumbar Disc Lesions
Card 3 - Reference Hospitalization and Follow-up

Case Number   1 2 3. 4 5

IV. Reference Hospitalization (continued)

C. Dates		D. Significant Hospital	E. Final Diagnosis		F. Therapy
1. Month	2. Year	Admission (do not code)	HNP – Location	Other Dx	1. Conservative
01 Jan 05 May 09 Sep	Last two		1 L-1 – L-2		a. Type
02 Feb 06 June 10 Oct	digits	Day Month Year	2 L-2 – L-3		0 None
03 Mar 07 July 11 Nov			3 L-3 – L-4		1 Bed rest
04 Apr 08 Aug 12 Dec	VV Unknown		4 L-4 – L-5		2 Lumbosacral belt
VV Unknown		_____ _____ _____	5 L-5 – S-1		3 Physiotherapy
			6 Other –		4 Postural exercises
		Name-	V Unknown		5 Manipulation
	6 7 8 9				6 Leg traction
Admission			Side		7 Procaine or
	10 11 12 13		7 Right		other injection
Reference			8 Left		8 Brace or body cast
Date			9 Bilateral		9 Other –
	14 15 16 17	18	19	20 21 22	V Unknown
Discharge					23

IV Reference Hospitalization
F. Therapy
2. Surgical

c. Date of Operation		d. Anesthesia		e. Operative Findings	f. Location of Findings	g. Relation to Myelogram
1. Month	2. Year	1. Type	2. Associated Complications	0 Normal	0 No abn.	0 No myelogram
Same as	Last two	1 Spinal		1 Herniated nucleus	Abn. between	1 Both positive,
cols. 6 - 7	digits	2 General	0 None	2 "Free fragment"	1 L-1 – L-2	same level
		3 Local	1 Infection	3 "Concealed disc"	2 L-2 – L-3	2 Both positive,
	VV Unknown	4 Combination	2 Paraplegia	4 Midline protrusion	3 L-3 – L-4	diff. level
		9 Other –	3 Death	5 Undue vert. mobility	4 L-4 – L-5	3 Both positive,
Day Month Year		V Unknown	9 Other –	6 Thick. ligamentum	5 L-5 – S-1	level unspec.
			V Unknown	flavum	6 Other –	4 Both negative
				7 Excessive extradural	V Unknown	5 Myelo. pos.,
				veins	DP	oper. neg.
				9 Other –	7 Right	6 Myelo. neg.,
				V Unknown	8 Left	oper. pos.
____ ____ ____					9 Bilateral	V Unknown
30 31	32 33	34	35	36	37	38

V Summary of Hosp., Operations and HNP Diagnoses (Do not include RH)

VI VA Compensation

B. Operations				C. Diagnoses of HNP	A. 1 Year after Discharge	B. At Cut-off
1. Total	2. Type of Procedure	3. Findings	4. Location of Findings			
X None (omit thru 53)	0 >1 oper. at same level	Same as col. 36	Same as col. 37	0 None	0 In service	
1 1				1 – 9 and V	1 No claim filed	
2 2	1 – 9 and V			same as col. 19	2 Claim disallowed (include 0%)	
etc.	same as col. 27				3 Rated, 10 – 20 %	
9 ≥ 9					4 " , 30 – 40 %	
V Unknown					5 " , 50 – 60 %	
					6 " , 70 – 80 %	
					7 " , 90 – 100 %	
					8 Rec. retirement pay	
					9 NSC pension from VA	
					V Unknown status or %	
					X DP – Died prior to date	
					Discharge _____	
					Total	HNP or rel. cond.	Total	HNP or rel. cond.
50	51	52	53	54	55	56	57	58

Name _____

NAS–NRC
FUA R20–8 Rev
June 1961

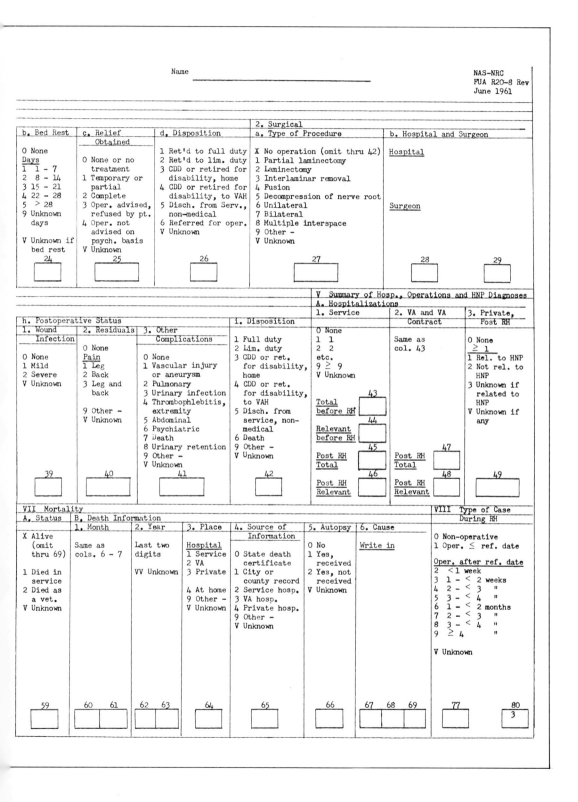

b. Bed Rest	c. Relief Obtained	d. Disposition	2. Surgical a. Type of Procedure	b. Hospital and Surgeon
0 None Days 1 1 - 7 2 8 - 14 3 15 - 21 4 22 - 28 5 > 28 9 Unknown days V Unknown if bed rest	0 None or no treatment 1 Temporary or partial 2 Complete 3 Oper. advised, refused by pt. 4 Oper. not advised on psych. basis V Unknown	1 Ret'd to full duty 2 Ret'd to lim. duty 3 CDD or retired for disability, home 4 CDD or retired for disability, to VAH 5 Disch. from Serv., non–medical 6 Referred for oper. V Unknown	X No operation (omit thru 42) 1 Partial laminectomy 2 Laminectomy 3 Interlaminar removal 4 Fusion 5 Decompression of nerve root 6 Unilateral 7 Bilateral 8 Multiple interspace 9 Other – V Unknown	Hospital

Surgeon |
| 24 | 25 | 26 | 27 | 28   29 |

V Summary of Hosp., Operations and HNP Diagnoses
A. Hospitalizations

h. Postoperative Status			i. Disposition	1. Service	2. VA and VA Contract	3. Private, Post RH
1. Wound Infection	2. Residuals	3. Other Complications		0 None 1 1 2 2 etc. 9 ≥ 9 V Unknown	Same as col. 43	0 None ≥ 1 1 Rel. to HNP 2 Not rel. to HNP 3 Unknown if related to HNP V Unknown if any
0 None 1 Mild 2 Severe V Unknown	0 None Pain 1 Leg 2 Back 3 Leg and back 9 Other – V Unknown	0 None 1 Vascular injury or aneurysm 2 Pulmonary 3 Urinary infection 4 Thrombophlebitis, extremity 5 Abdominal 6 Psychiatric 7 Death 8 Urinary retention 9 Other – V Unknown	1 Full duty 2 Lim. duty 3 CDD or ret. for disability, home 4 CDD or ret. for disability, to VAH 5 Disch. from service, non– medical 6 Death 9 Other – V Unknown	Total before RH 44 Relevant before RH 45 Post RH Total 46 Post RH Relevant	Post RH Total 48 Post RH Relevant	
39	40	41	42	43	47	49

VII Mortality							VIII Type of Case During RH
A. Status	B. Death Information						
	1. Month	2. Year	3. Place	4. Source of Information	5. Autopsy	6. Cause	
X Alive (omit thru 69) 1 Died in service 2 Died as a vet. V Unknown	Same as cols. 6 - 7	Last two digits VV Unknown	Hospital 1 Service 2 VA 3 Private 4 At home 9 Other – V Unknown	0 State death certificate 1 City or county record 2 Service hosp. 3 VA hosp. 4 Private hosp. 9 Other – V Unknown	0 No 1 Yes, received 2 Yes, not received V Unknown	Write in	0 Non-operative 1 Oper. ≤ ref. date Oper. after ref. date 2 <1 week 3 1 - < 2 weeks 4 2 - < 3 " 5 3 - < 4 " 6 1 - < 2 months 7 2 - < 3 " 8 3 - < 4 " 9 ≥ 4 " V Unknown
59	60 61	62 63	64	65	66	67 68 69	77 80 3

Form FUA R20–9

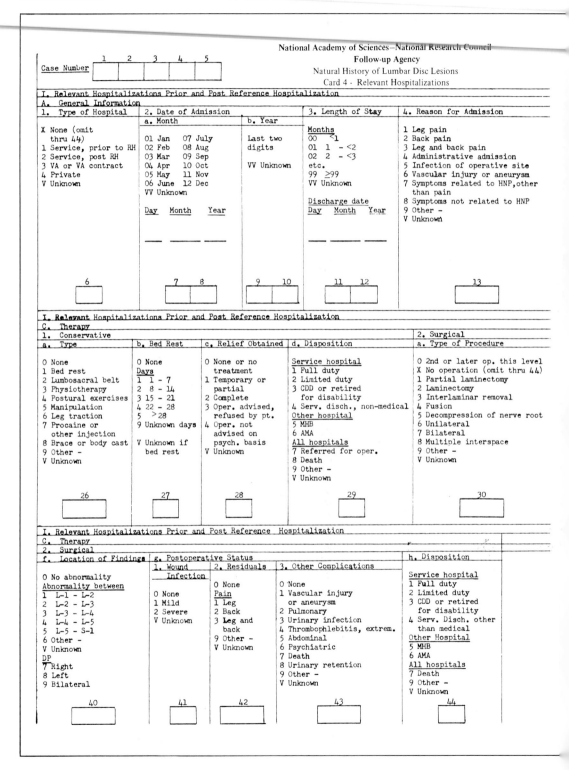

National Academy of Sciences–National Research Council
Follow-up Agency
Natural History of Lumbar Disc Lesions
Card 4 - Relevant Hospitalizations

Case Number 1 2 3 4 5

I. Relevant Hospitalizations Prior and Post Reference Hospitalization
A. General Information

1. Type of Hospital	2. Date of Admission		3. Length of Stay	4. Reason for Admission
	a. Month	b. Year		
X None (omit thru 44)	01 Jan 07 July	Last two digits	Months	1 Leg pain
1 Service, prior to RH	02 Feb 08 Aug		00 <1	2 Back pain
2 Service, post RH	03 Mar 09 Sep	VV Unknown	01 1 - <2	3 Leg and back pain
3 VA or VA contract	04 Apr 10 Oct		02 2 - <3	4 Administrative admission
4 Private	05 May 11 Nov		etc.	5 Infection of operative site
V Unknown	06 June 12 Dec		99 >99	6 Vascular injury or aneurysm
	VV Unknown		VV Unknown	7 Symptoms related to HNP, other than pain
	Day Month Year		Discharge date	8 Symptoms not related to HNP
	___ ___ ___		Day Month Year	9 Other –
			___ ___ ___	V Unknown
6	7 8	9 10	11 12	13

I. Relevant Hospitalizations Prior and Post Reference Hospitalization
C. Therapy

1. Conservative				2. Surgical
a. Type	b. Bed Rest	c. Relief Obtained	d. Disposition	a. Type of Procedure
0 None	0 None	0 None or no treatment	Service hospital	0 2nd or later op. this level
1 Bed rest	Days		1 Full duty	X No operation (omit thru 44)
2 Lumbosacral belt	1 1 - 7	1 Temporary or partial	2 Limited duty	1 Partial laminectomy
3 Physiotherapy	2 8 - 14		3 CDD or retired for disability	2 Laminectomy
4 Postural exercises	3 15 - 21	2 Complete	4 Serv. disch., non-medical	3 Interlaminar removal
5 Manipulation	4 22 - 28	3 Oper. advised, refused by pt.	Other hospital	4 Fusion
6 Leg traction	5 >28		5 MHB	5 Decompression of nerve root
7 Procaine or other injection	9 Unknown days	4 Oper. not advised on psych. basis	6 AMA	6 Unilateral
8 Brace or body cast	V Unknown if bed rest	V Unknown	All hospitals	7 Bilateral
9 Other –			7 Referred for oper.	8 Multiple interspace
V Unknown			8 Death	9 Other –
			9 Other –	V Unknown
			V Unknown	
26	27	28	29	30

I. Relevant Hospitalizations Prior and Post Reference Hospitalization
C. Therapy
2. Surgical

f. Location of Findings	g. Postoperative Status			h. Disposition
	1. Wound Infection	2. Residuals	3. Other Complications	
0 No abnormality	0 None	0 None	0 None	Service hospital
Abnormality between	1 Mild	Pain	1 Vascular injury or aneurysm	1 Full duty
1 L-1 - L-2	2 Severe	1 Leg	2 Pulmonary	2 Limited duty
2 L-2 - L-3	V Unknown	2 Back	3 Urinary infection	3 CDD or retired for disability
3 L-3 - L-4		3 Leg and back	4 Thrombophlebitis, extrem.	4 Serv. Disch. other than medical
4 L-4 - L-5		9 Other –	5 Abdominal	Other Hospital
5 L-5 - S-1		V Unknown	6 Psychiatric	5 MHB
6 Other –			7 Death	6 AMA
V Unknown			8 Urinary retention	All hospitals
DP			9 Other –	7 Death
7 Right			V Unknown	9 Other –
8 Left				V Unknown
9 Bilateral				
40	41	42	43	44

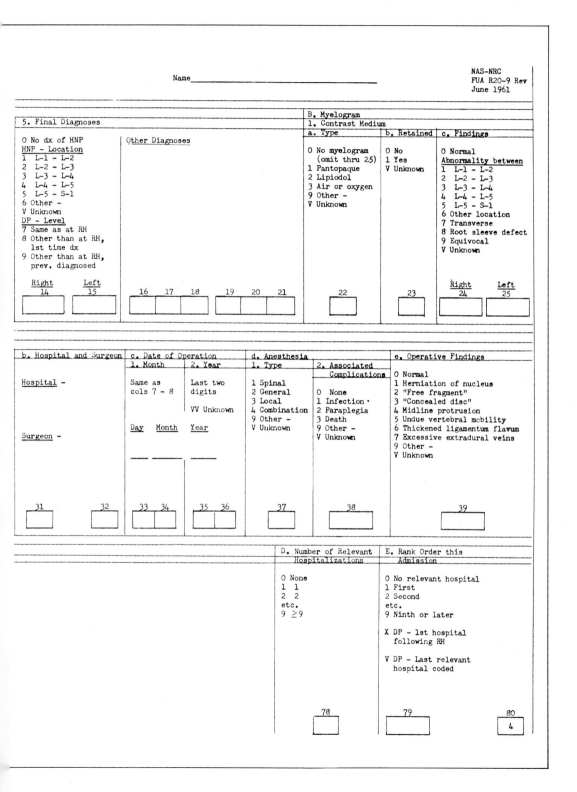

Name _____

NAS-NRC
FUA R20-9 Rev
June 1961

5. Final Diagnoses

O No dx of HNP
HNP - Location
1 L-1 - L-2
2 L-2 - L-3
3 L-3 - L-4
4 L-4 - L-5
5 L-5 - S-1
6 Other -
V Unknown
DP - Level
7 Same as at RH
8 Other than at RH,
   1st time dx
9 Other than at RH,
   prev. diagnosed

Other Diagnoses

|Right 14|Left 15|16|17|18|19|20|21|

B. Myelogram
1. Contrast Medium

a. Type

O No myelogram
   (omit thru 25)
1 Pantopaque
2 Lipiodol
3 Air or oxygen
9 Other -
V Unknown

b. Retained

O No
1 Yes
V Unknown

c. Findings

O Normal
Abnormality between
1 L-1 - L-2
2 L-2 - L-3
3 L-3 - L-4
4 L-4 - L-5
5 L-5 - S-1
6 Other location
7 Transverse
8 Root sleeve defect
9 Equivocal
V Unknown

|22|23|Right 24|Left 25|

---

b. Hospital and Surgeon

Hospital -

Surgeon -

|31|32|

c. Date of Operation

1. Month
Same as
cols 7 - 8

2. Year
Last two
digits

VV Unknown

Day   Month   Year

_____ _____ _____

|33 34|35 36|

d. Anesthesia

1. Type
1 Spinal
2 General
3 Local
4 Combination
9 Other -
V Unknown

2. Associated
   Complications
O None
1 Infection ·
2 Paraplegia
3 Death
9 Other -
V Unknown

|37|38|

e. Operative Findings

O Normal
1 Herniation of nucleus
2 "Free fragment"
3 "Concealed disc"
4 Midline protrusion
5 Undue vertebral mobility
6 Thickened ligamentum flavum
7 Excessive extradural veins
9 Other -
V Unknown

|39|

D. Number of Relevant Hospitalizations

O None
1 1
2 2
etc.
9 ≥ 9

E. Rank Order this Admission

O No relevant hospital
1 First
2 Second
etc.
9 Ninth or later

X DP - 1st hospital
  following RH

V DP - Last relevant
  hospital coded

|78|79|80|
| | | 4 |

ALLOCATION OF PATIENTS FOR FOLLOW-UP EXAMINATION, CASE CONTACTING, AND EXAMINATION PROCEDURE

The clinical investigators were furnished by the FUA with the following:

Copies of clinical records

Reference hospital roentgenograms, if available

Instructions regarding the contacting and examination of patients

Forms FUA R20-12 for recording status of patient contacting and reporting it to the FUA

Forms FUA R20-6a and 6b and Sensory Charts (Figs. 10 and 11) for recording the results of the examination

Letters to be used in contacting patients

Postcards for use by patients in scheduling examinations

The relevant materials follow and their use is described in the memorandum on Case Allocation, Contact, and Examination Procedures and in the Instructions for the Clinical Examination.

NATIONAL ACADEMY OF SCIENCES
NATIONAL RESEARCH COUNCIL

2101 CONSTITUTION AVENUE, WASHINGTON 25, D. C.

DIVISION OF MEDICAL SCIENCES

Follow-up Agency

15 January 1962

MEMORANDUM TO: Clinical Participants in the VA Cooperative Study of the Natural History of Lumbar Disc Lesions

FROM: M. Dean Nefzger

SUBJECT: Case Allocation, Contact, and Examination Procedures

1. When a case is ready for assignment, all pertinent material will be sent to the investigator responsible for the examination. This material has been systematically collected specifically for this study and should remain in the investigator's possession at all times until it is returned to the National Academy of Sciences–National Research Council. The following will be included:

    a. Abstract of medical history

    b. Photostats of selected clinical material

    c. Original Army x-ray films, if available

    d. Examination form to be completed by investigator

    e. Contact status report form

    f. Sensory chart

2. On receipt of these materials, the following procedures for contacting the veteran should be initiated:

    a. Standard letter 1, attached, should be sent by *certified mail* requesting a return receipt signed by the addressee only. This letter should be individually prepared on VA hospital stationery, and should include a preaddressed postal card suggesting alternative dates for the examination, which the veteran can complete and return to you. Such postal cards will be supplied, but will have to be addressed before used.

b. If your first letter is not returned or reply is not received within 2 weeks, send standard letter 2, attached, by regular mail. This also should be individually prepared on VA hospital stationery. If necessary, this letter may be slightly modified to fit special circumstances of the hospital or veteran.

c. If reply is not received within 2 weeks after sending standard letter 2, contact the man by telephone, telegram, or other means in an effort to persuade him to participate or to determine his reasons for refusing. It would be desirable to learn as much as possible about men who will not cooperate, especially from the standpoint of apparent physical health. It may even be possible to have a social worker visit the homes of such men.

3. Since addresses are taken, without verification, from records, some are certain to be incorrect. If an address is incorrect, the first letter sent by certified mail will be returned to you. If you are unable to locate the correct address, notify the National Academy of Sciences–National Research Council on the contact status report form and tracing procedures will be initiated here. Do *not* send the veteran's case material to us at this time. To minimize shipments and consequent losses, case material should be retained in the hospital until requested or until a new address is furnished. When the veteran is located, we will send his address to you, and contact procedures may be instituted again.

4. When contact with the veteran has been made, we should be notified of the result on the contact status report form. If an appointment for examination is set, show the date, or if an appointment cannot be made, give the reason. If the veteran cannot be reached, we should be notified on the contract status report form within 30 days of the date of allocation.

5. Appropriate administrative arrangements should be made in advance so that the veteran can report directly to the responsible investigator soon after his arrival at the hospital. In addition to your interview and examination, the veteran should be referred for the necessary x-ray films. AP, lateral, and oblique views of the lumbosacral area should be taken with the veteran recumbent. In addition, bending x-ray films should be taken of all men with fusions as follows:

Extension: Veteran will stand erect in a lateral position with a satisfactory coverage of the 14×17 film centering in the midpoint between the lumbosacral joint and T12-L1. He will extend the maximal allowable degree.

Flexion: Veteran will stand erect laterally, bend forward with the knees fully extended, and grasp the legs as far distally as possible.

Lateral bending: Veteran will flex laterally carrying the palm of the hand down the side of the leg with the knees fully extended. Repeat both left and right.

6. Detailed instructions and definitions for the examination form will be distributed separately. Study forms should be carefully completed and reviewed by the responsible investigator and returned, together with all x-ray films (Army and VA) and other case material, to the National Academy of Sciences–National Research Council by *certified mail.* Every precaution should be observed to insure that information obtained by interview, examination, and x-ray plates or reports does *not* get into the veteran's hospital record or claims folder. If it is necessary to prepare standard VA forms for local administrative purposes, these should indicate only that the veteran was seen, examined, or x-rayed.

MDN/fw
Enclosures

(Standard letter 1)

Dear Mr. _____:

Your help is needed in an important new study that is being conducted by the Veterans Administration and the National Academy of Sciences–National Research Council. Our medical records show that you are one of many veterans who suffered with low back difficulties while in the Armed Forces, and we are interested in a complete evaluation of your present health to better understand your condition. It is hoped that this research will provide some of the information needed to determine the causes of these conditions, to prevent their occurrence in others, and to improve present methods of treatment.

Your disability rating, compensation, or pension will not be reduced as a result of participation. The information is confidential and will be used for research purposes only.

The purpose of this letter is to request you to report to this hospital so that I may review your medical history with you and make the examinations and tests necessary for a full evaluation of your present health. Your visit will be scheduled to suit your convenience. If you arrive at the hospital during the early morning, every effort will be made to finish in one day. You will be reimbursed for the cost of round-trip travel.

I sincerely hope you are able to take advantage of this opportunity and that you will agree to participate with me in this undertaking. Enclosed is a postal card that you may use in replying to this letter. Please give the specific dates on which you would prefer an appointment.

Sincerely,

_____

Enclosure

(Standard letter 2)

Dear Mr. _____:

I wrote you recently about participation in a study of men who suffered from back pain during service in the Army. Since I have not received your reply, I am again writing to urge your cooperation. I would like to emphasize that it is important to know about your present health, regardless of whether you now have trouble with your back.

The sole purpose of this research is to learn as much as possible about the causes, prevention, and best treatment of back pain. The needed information can be obtained only by examining men like you who have been hospitalized with back trouble. A great deal can be learned in this way, but only if everyone selected for study extends his full cooperation.

Your help will be greatly appreciated and will represent a significant contribution to medical science. You may be sure that the confidential information obtained during this examination will not alter your compensation status in any way.

A preaddressed postal card is enclosed for your convenience. Please indicate the date and time that would be most convenient for you to come to the hospital for examination. Transportation costs to and from the hospital will be reimbursed.

Sincerely,

_____

Enclosure

VA COOPERATIVE STUDY OF THE NATURAL HISTORY
OF LUMBAR DISC LESIONS

Instructions for Use of Forms FUA R20-6a and 6b
Clinical Examination

Forms 6a and 6b constitute the record of historical and clinical findings obtained directly from the veteran at the time of interview and examination by a participating physician. Information may be recorded on these forms by circling the number of the appropriate category or by checking or writing in the appropriate item box. Every item has been designed to require an answer even if only to indicate that a condition is not present or that pertinent information is unknown. If the space provided is not sufficient for all pertinent information, your comment may be continued on the back of the sheet.

When completed, these forms, all x-ray films, and all other case materials should be returned, in one package, to the Follow-up Agency, National Academy of Sciences–National Research Council. Following is a detailed description of the desired information, how it should be obtained, and how recorded.

Form FUA R20-6a
item number   **Instructions**

I. **General information**

   A. *Examiner and hospital*

      Write in the appropriate space the name of the hospital where examination was performed. The examiner should sign his name after the form has been reviewed to indicate that it is complete and correct.

   B. *Date of examination*

      The date of the examination (day, month, and year) should be entered in the space provided.

II. **History**

   A. *Family history*

    1. Sciatica
    2. Low back pain
    3. Operations for ruptured lumbar disc
    4. Operations for ruptured cervical or thoracic discs

      In the appropriate box on the form, circle any one or combination of numbers to indicate a history of the above conditions among relatives of the veteran. If more than one brother or more than one sister is involved, give the number of each.

      When using item 4, operations for ruptured cervical or thoracic discs, write in the area involved. If a disc operation has been performed but it is not known in which area, indicate which relative was involved under item 4 and circle the X to indicate uncertainty as to area.

      In these items the V should be circled when it is not known which relative had the specified condition. Whenever the position ⌐, other, is circled, the relationship should be specified, that is, uncle, aunt, cousin, etc.

   B. *Patient's adult medical history*

    1. Cervical disc rupture
    2. Thoracic disc rupture

Continued.

Instructions for use of Form FUA R20–6a—cont'd

3. Spontaneous compression of median or ulnar nerve

4. Hypertrophic osteoarthritis
5. Marie-Strumpell arthritis
6. Bursitis
7. Periarticular fibrosis or calcification
8. Shoulder-arm syndrome
9. Hip disease
10. Periarteritis
11. Keloid formation
12. Other neoplastic disease
13. Urinary calculi or other renal disease
14. Parasitic disease
15. Infections (severe, chronic, or repetitive)
16. Other
    Indicate whether the veteran has ever had or now has any of the above items by checking "yes," "no," or "unknown" on the form. For items 12 through 16 specific diagnosis should be given, and for every item the date of onset should be written in.

C. *Present residuals of disc disability*
    Circle at least one number to indicate the veteran's present complaints representing residuals of previous disc rupture. If position 9, other residual disc disability, is used, the specific condition should be given. If the veteran has sensory complaints, indicate the type, degree, and location of the abnormality.

D. *Occupational history*
    1. Preservice occupation
       Write in the veteran's immediate preservice occupation (i.e., carpenter, laborer, store manager, lawyer, student), the industry in which he was engaged (i.e., construction, manufacturing, transportation, personal services, professional services), and the dates or duration of that employment.
    2. Immediately after discharge
       Write in the occupation and industry of the veteran's first employment after discharge from the Army following World War II, and give the date or duration of this employment. Unemployment should be entered only if the veteran was unable to find suitable work because of disability. If the veteran was unable to find employment, give the specific reason. Reentry to the Armed Forces may be recorded as an occupation.
    3. Present employment
       Write in the veteran's present occupation, the industry of his employer, and the dates or duration of this employment.
    4. Activity in present occupation
       By circling the appropriate number, indicate the amount of activity required of the veteran in his present occupation. If the veteran feels that he is not fully able to meet the demands of this present occupation, the X also should be circled to indicate a limitation.
    5. Reason for occupational change
       If the veteran's employment status has changed, or if he has changed jobs since discharge from the Army, determine whether these changes reflect physical limitations resulting from the previous disc rupture. If there have been no occupational changes, other than the normal progression expected over 15 years, the O position should be used. The V position should be used only to indicate that it is not known whether occupational changes have occurred.

Form FUA R20-6b
item number   **Instructions**

III. **Examination** (page 2)

    A. *Back*

        1. General findings

            Circle any one or any combination of numbers to record observed general abnormalities of the back. If position 3, other abnormalities, is used, write in the specific finding.

            Paravertebral muscle spasm, position 2, is defined as a reactive muscle contracture unrelieved by a rest posture for that muscle. For example, lumbar paravertebral muscle spasm should be relieved by hyperextension or by putting the veteran in a prone position. If paravertebral muscle spasm is unrelieved in either of these positions, position 2 should be circled. If the spasm is relieved, position 2 should not be circled.

        2. Lumbar scoliosis

          a. Standing

          b. Lying

            Convexity to the right means that the curvature in the lumbar region is toward the veteran's right side. Alternating scoliosis should be recorded when the veteran can voluntarily change the curvature from one side to the other but cannot maintain the spine in a straight position.

        3. Localized tenderness

        4. Localized percussion

            Perform localized percussion of spinous processes with a reflex hammer.

        5. Jugular compression

            With the veteran in a supine position, compress jugular veins in neck for 5 to 10 seconds, using a firm pressure of hands. Reinforcement with abdominal straining may be used. A positive result is indicated by pain in the back or legs.

        6. Spinal movement from neutral position

          a. Flexion

          b. Extension

          c. Lateral flexion (right and left)

          d. Rotation (right and left)

            These measurements should be made by goniometer following the instructions set forth by the AMA Committee on Medical Rating of Physical Impairment, A Guide to the Evaluation of Permanent Impairment of the Extremities and Back, J.A.M.A., February 15, 1958. Pages 96, 98, and 100 of this special issue are attached here for easy reference.* It should be noted whether the spinal movements are associated with subjective pain, whether flexion is from the hip joints, and whether the lumbar spine arches normally.

    B. *Lower extremities*

        1. Straight leg raising (right and left)

            With patient in a supine position on a flat table, use a goniometer to measure the angle through which each leg separately can be raised with the knee extended. Consider the horizontal plane of the table as zero degrees.

---

*See pp. 87 to 91 and Figs. 1 to 7.   *Continued.*

Instructions for use of Form FUA R20–6b—cont'd

2. Sciatic tenderness (right and left)

Palpate the course of the sciatic nerve in the thigh, buttock, and popliteal fossa with the patient in the prone position.

3. Gait

For this purpose limp shall be the equivalent of functional disability, that is, "limp, right" means there is a functional disability of the right leg that contributes to an uneven or irregular gait.

4. Muscle strength

Test each indicated muscle group by having the patient exert force against the examiner's hand while in a supine position.

5. Thigh and calf circumferences

With patient supine and legs straight, measure the circumference of the thigh at a point 15 cm. above the superior border of the patella. Look for the maximum circumference of the largest calf, and measure both legs at that level. Record all measurements to the nearest centimeter.

6. Decreased sensation to pain and touch (right and left)

Use a sharp pin to test sensitivity to pain and a wisp of cotton to test touch. By comparing one limb with the other, determine sensory dermatomes of decreased or increased sensitivity. Outline the sensory changes involved on the special forms provided for this purpose and attach to this examination form (Figs. 10 and 11). Attached to these instructions is a figure showing dermatomes (Figs. 8 and 9).

7. Hyperalgesia or hyperpathia (right and left)

Indicate the presence, absence, or aberration of sensation as above detected by testing or reported by patient. Outline the sensory area involved on the sensory chart (Figs. 10 and 11).

8. Tendon reflexes

Test knee jerks with patient in the supine position, and ankle jerks with patient in prone position.

IV. **Evaluation**

A. *Use of back*

If there is a noticeable limitation in the use of the back, determine and record the reason for this. If position 4, other, is used, write in the specific reason.

To use position 9, adverse functional overlay, it will be necessary to determine whether the limitation is wholly structural or whether it is in part functional. Use position 9 only if there is a significant functional component.

B. *Use of lower extremities*

Indicate the extent of loss of use of legs.

C. *Employment*

If the veteran feels he is not fully able to work, attempt a characterization of the extent of this limitation.

D. *Examiner's overall functional impression*

This evaluation should take into account all the physical and psychogenic factors, as judged by the present examiner, that might be involved in the veteran's disc disease at the time of examination. The examiner should indicate the answers with a brief general statement of his overall impression plus indicating the amount of involvement as 0-25, 25-50, 50-75, or 75-100.

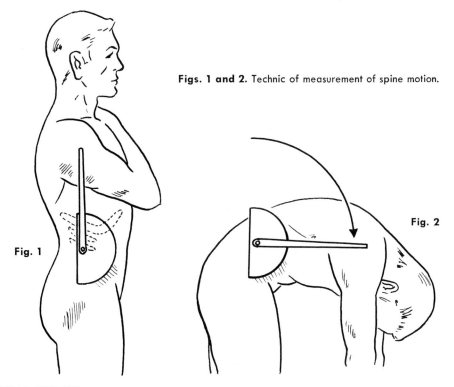

Figs. 1 and 2. Technic of measurement of spine motion.

Fig. 1

Fig. 2

DORSOLUMBAR REGION*
Technic of measurement: flexion—extension
Restricted motion

1. Place patient in neutral position as shown in Fig. 1. Arm is raised in figure merely to show placement of goniometer.
2. Center goniometer along mid-axillary line at level of lowest rib as shown in Fig. 1. Record goniometer reading.
3. *Flexion:* With patient bending as far forward as possible as shown in Fig. 2, follow range of motion, keeping goniometer arm along mid-axillary line. Note goniometer base is to be kept in line with femur. Record end of arc of motion.
4. *Extension:* Starting from neutral position with patient bending as far backward as possible, follow range of motion with goniometer arm. Record end of arc of motion.
5. Consult Restricted Motion Table† for corresponding impairment of spine. *Example:* 20 degrees active flexion from neutral position (0°) or any 20 degree arc of retained active flexion = 7% impairment of spine.
6. Add spine impairment values contributed by flexion and extension. The sum of these values is impairment of spine contributed by flexion and extension of dorsolumbar region.

*From Committee of Medical Rating of Physical Impairment: A guide to the evaluation of permanent impairment of the extremities and back, J.A.M.A. (special issue), pp. 96, 98, 100, Feb. 15, 1958.
†This table was not used in the present study.

Ankylosis

1. Place goniometer base as if measuring neutral position shown above. Measure deviation from neutral position with goniometer arm. Record goniometer reading.

2. Consult Ankylosis Table for Dorsolumbar Region* for corresponding impairment of spine.

   Example: Dorsolumbar region ankylosed at 20 degrees flexion = 37% impairment of spine.

or

1. Determine number and position of ankylosed vertebrae by appropriate x-ray methods.

2. Consult appropriate Ankylosis Table for Vertebrae* for corresponding impairment of spine.

Technic of measurement: lateral flexion

Restricted motion

1. Place patient in neutral position as shown in Fig. 3.

2. Center goniometer as shown in Fig. 3 with base over posterior superior iliac spines and goniometer arm along midline of back. Record goniometer reading.

3. *Left lateral flexion:* With patient bending to left as far as possible as shown in Fig. 4, follow range of motion with goniometer arm. Record end of arc of motion.

4. *Right lateral flexion:* Starting from neutral position with patient bending to right as far as possible as shown in Fig. 5, follow range of motion with goniometer arm. Record end of arc of motion.

5. Consult Restricted Motion Table* for corresponding impairment of spine.

   Example: 10 degrees active left lateral flexion from neutral position (0°) or any 10 degree arc of retained left lateral flexion = 2% impairment of spine.

---

*This table was not used in the present study.

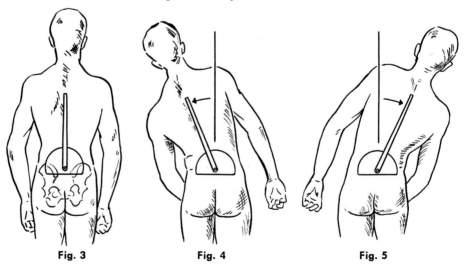

Fig. 3   Fig. 4   Fig. 5

6. Add spine impairment values as contributed by left lateral flexion and right lateral flexion. The sum of these values is impairment of spine contributed by lateral flexion of dorsolumbar region.

Ankylosis

1. Place goniometer base as if measuring neutral position shown above. Measure deviation from neutral position with goniometer arm. Record goniometer reading.
2. Consult Ankylosis Table for Dorsolumbar Region* for corresponding impairment of spine.
    Example: Dorsolumbar region ankylosed at 10 degrees right lateral flexion = 45% impairment of spine.

or

1. Determine number and position of ankylosed vertebrae by appropriate x-ray methods.
2. Consult appropriate Ankylosis Table for Vertebrae* for corresponding impairment of spine.

Technic of measurement: rotation

Restricted motion

1. Place patient in neutral position as shown in Fig. 6, with examiner preventing motion of pelvis. The goniometer is not used.
2. With patient twisting to right and left as far as possible as shown in Fig. 7,

---

*This table was not used in the present study.

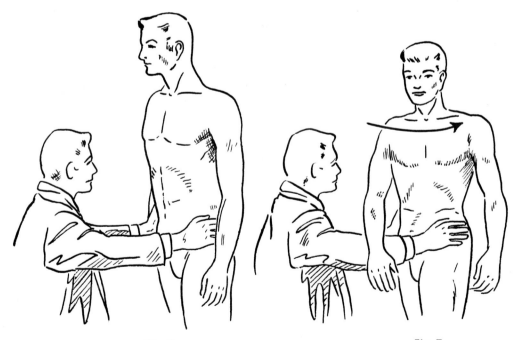

Fig. 6   Fig. 7

record range of motion in each direction *separately* as estimated by arc described by frontal plane of body as it turns from neutral position.

3. Consult Restricted Motion Table* for corresponding impairment of spine. *Example:* 10 degrees active left rotation from neutral position (0°) or any 10 degree arc of retained active left rotation = 4% impairment of spine.

4. Add spine impairment values contributed by left rotation and right rotation. The sum of these values is impairment of spine contributed by rotation of dorsolumbar region.

———

*This table was not used in the present study.

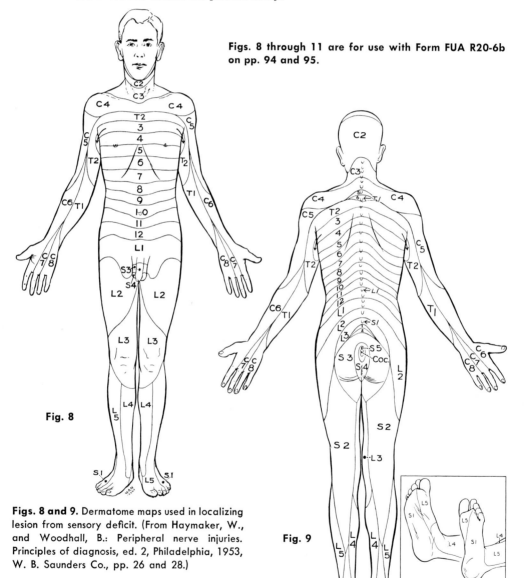

Figs. 8 through 11 are for use with Form FUA R20-6b on pp. 94 and 95.

Fig. 8

Fig. 9

Figs. 8 and 9. Dermatome maps used in localizing lesion from sensory deficit. (From Haymaker, W., and Woodhall, B.: Peripheral nerve injuries. Principles of diagnosis, ed. 2, Philadelphia, 1953, W. B. Saunders Co., pp. 26 and 28.)

Ankylosis

1. Estimate and record angle at which dorsolumbar region is ankylosed by position of frontal plane of body.
2. Consult Ankylosis Table for Dorsolumbar Region* for corresponding impairment of spine.
   Example: Dorsolumbar region ankylosed at 10 degrees right rotation = 40% impairment of spine.

or

1. Determine number and position of ankylosed vertebrae by appropriate x-ray methods.
2. Consult appropriate Ankylosis Table for Vertebrae* for corresponding impairment of spine.

---

*This table was not used in the present study.

HERNIATED DISC STUDY
Sensory chart—anterior

Name _____ Date _____ No. _____

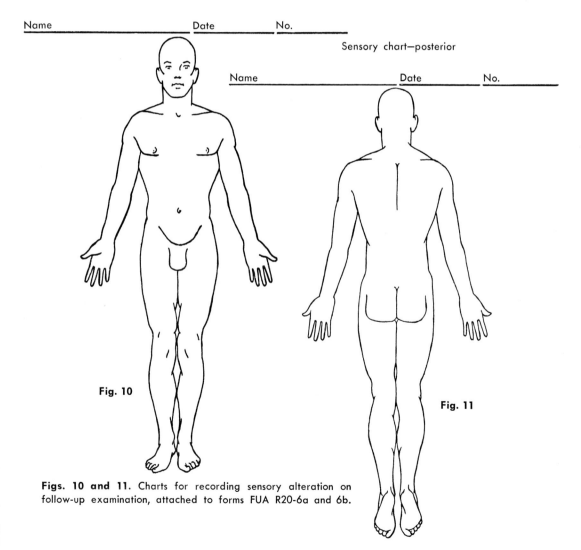

Sensory chart—posterior

Name _____ Date _____ No. _____

Fig. 10

Fig. 11

Figs. 10 and 11. Charts for recording sensory alteration on follow-up examination, attached to forms FUA R20-6a and 6b.

Form FUA R20–6a

Case Number [1] [2] [3] [4] [5]

National Academy of Sciences–National Research Council
Follow-up Agency
Natural History of Lumbar Disc Lesions
Page 1 - Examination

I General Information

A. Examiner and Hospital where Examined

Hospital

_____

Signature of Examiner

_____

_____

B. Date of Examination

Day   Month   Year

_____

II History

A. Family

1. Sciatica	2. Low Back Pain
0 None	0 None
1 Father	1 Father
2 Mother	2 Mother
3 Brother	3 Brother
4 Sister	4 Sister
5 Other –	5 Other –
V Unknown	V Unknown

II History

B. Patient's Adult Medical History

	No	Yes	Unknown	Comments (Dates etc.)		
1. Cervical disc rupture					9. Hip disease	
2. Thoracic disc rupture					10. Periarteritis	
3. Spontaneous compression of median or ulnar nerve					11. Keloid formation	
4. Hypertrophic osteoarthritis					12. Neoplastic disease	
5. Marie–Strumpell arthritis					13. Urinary calculi or other renal disease	
6. Bursitis					14. Parasitic disease	
7. Periarticular fibrosis or calcification					15. Infections (severe, chronic or repetitive)	
8. Shoulder-arm syndrome					16. Other –	

III History

D. Employment

	1. Preservice	2. Immediately after Discharge	3. Present
Occupation			
Nature of Employer's Business			
Duration or Dates			

Name _____

NAS-NRC
FUA R20-6a Rev
Sept 1961

3. Operations for Ruptured Lumbar Disc	4. Operations for Ruptured Cervical and Thoracic Disc
0 None	0 None
1 Father	1 Father
2 Mother	2 Mother
3 Brother	3 Brother
4 Sister	4 Sister
5 Other -	5 Other -
	V Unknown
V Unknown	X Disc operation performed, area unknown

No	Yes	Unknown	Comments (Dates etc.)	C. Present Residuals of Disc Disability
				0 None
				1 Mild intermittent low back pain
				2 Mod. " " " "
				3 Severe " " " "
				4 Mild recurrent sciatica
				5 Mod. " "
				6 Severe " "
				7 Urinary sphincter disturbance
				8 Rectal " "
				9 Other disc disability -
				V Unknown

4. Activity in Present Occupation	5. Change in Occupation
1 Sedentary	0 No change made
2 Light labor	1 Employed now, not previously
3 Heavy labor	2 Changed because of disc injury
4 Other -	3 Changed for other reason
	4 Changed, reason unknown
	5 Unemployed because of disc injury
	6 Unemployed for other reason
V Unknown	7 Unemployed, reason unknown
X Limited in present job	V Unknown if occupation changed

Form FUA R20–6b

Case Number | 1 | 2 | 3 | 4 | 5

III Examination

A. Back

1. General Findings	2. Lumbar Scoliosis		3. Localized Tenderness	4. Localized Percussion	5. Jugular Compression
	a. Standing	b. Lying on Abd.			
0 Normal	0 None	0 None	0 None	0 None	0 No response
1 Loss of lumbar lordosis	1 Convex to right	1 Convex to right	1 Area of incision	Abnormal	1 Back pain
2 Paravertebral muscle spasm	2 Convex to left	2 Convex to left	2 Paravertebral with radiation	1 Cervical	2 Right leg pain
3 Other –	3 Alternating	3 Alternating	3 Paravertebral without radiation	2 Dorsal	3 Left leg pain
	4 Other –	4 Other –	4 Sacro-iliac	3 Lumbar	V Unknown or not done
			5 Other –	4 Sacral	
V Unknown	V Unknown	V Unknown	V Unknown	V Unknown or not done	

III Examination

B. Lower Extremities

4. Muscle Strength (Check appropriate spaces)

	Dorsal ext.,foot		Plantar ext.,foot		Ext. hallucis longus		Quadriceps femoris		Gluteal muscles	
	Right	Left	Right	Left	Right	Left	Right	Left	Right	Left
Normal										
Mild weakness										
Mod. weakness										
Severe weakness										
Unknown										
Visible contraction										

III Examination

B. Lower Extremities

8. Tendon Reflexes

	Ankle		Knee	
	Right	Left	Right	Left
0 Normal				
1 Increased				
2 Decreased				
3 Absent				
V Unknown				

IV Evaluation

A. Use of Back

0 Normal

Limited by

1 Pain

2 Weakness

3 Deformity

4 Other –

V Unknown

9 Adverse functional overlay

B. Use of Lower Extremities

0 Normal

1 Unlimited walking, cannot run

2 Walks less than 1/4 mile

3 Walks less than 1 block

4 Will not bear weight

5 Amputation, right leg

6 Amputation, left leg

7 Other –

V Unknown

Name _____

NAS—NRC
FUA R20—6b Rev
Sept 1961

6. Spinal Movement from Neutral Position, 0°)	B. Lower Extremities		
	1. Straight Leg-raising	2. Sciatic Tenderness	3. Gait

6. Spinal Movement from Neutral Position, 0°)	1. Straight Leg-raising	2. Sciatic Tenderness		3. Gait
a. Flexion _____ °	**Right**	**Right**	**Left**	0 Normal
b. Extension _____ °	0 Negative	0 None	0 None	1 Limp, right
c. Lateral flexion	Positive at _____ °	1 Sciatic notch	1 Sciatic notch	2 Limp, left
Right _____ °		2 Popliteal fossa	2 Popliteal fossa	3 Other –
Left _____ °	**Left**	3 Other –	3 Other –	
	0 Negative			
d. Rotation	Positive at _____ °			
Right _____ °				
Left _____ °		V Unknown	V Unknown	V Unknown

5. Thigh and Calf Circumferences	6. Decreased Sensation to Pain and Touch		7. Hyperalgesia	
Right thigh _____	**Right**	**Left**	**Right**	**Left**
	0 None	0 None	0 None	0 None
Left thigh _____	Dermatome	Dermatome	Dermatome	Dermatome
	1 L–4	1 L–4	1 L–4	1 L–4
Right calf _____	2 L–5	2 L–5	2 L–5	2 L–5
	3 S–1	3 S–1	3 S–1	3 S–1
	4 S–3,4,5	4 S–3,4,5	4 S–3,4,5	4 S–3,4,5
Left calf _____	5 Other –	5 Other –	5 Other –	5 Other –
	V Unknown	V Unknown	V Unknown	V Unknown

C. Employment	D. Examiner's Overall Functional Impression
0 No handicap apparent	0 No disability
1 Some handicap, not severe	
2 Severe handicap	
3 Man regards self as unemployable	Disability _____ %
4 Other –	
	V Unknown
V Unknown	

Patient's name_____   Hospital_____

Study number_____

NATURAL HISTORY OF LUMBAR DISC LESIONS
Contact Status Report

Mail contact

First letter sent (give date)_____
Reply received (give date)_____
Letter returned (give date)_____

Second letter sent (give date)_____
Reply received (give date)_____
Letter returned (give date)_____

Telephone contact

Date attempted_____ Successful? Yes____ No____
Date attempted_____ Successful? Yes____ No____
Date attempted_____ Successful? Yes____ No____

(see other side please)

NAS-NRC
FUA R20-12
Aug. 1961

Other contact attempts

Date_____ Method_____ Successful? Yes___ No___
Date_____ Method_____ Successful? Yes___ No___
Date_____ Method_____ Successful? Yes___ No___

Contact results

☐ Appointment accepted (give date set)_____
☐ Appointment refused (give reason):

Remarks:

Dear Doctor:

I have received your letter concerning an examination, and I will be able to keep an appointment on either of the following days:

_____ or _____
Day   Month   Year   Day   Month   Year

Thank you.

_____
(Name)

_____
(Address)

_____
(Telephone)

FOLLOW-UP REVIEW OF RADIOGRAPHIC MATERIALS

A committee of VA radiologists was formed and its members reviewed the available films. The materials sent to them consisted of the following:

Available roentgenograms of the lumbar spine and myelograms obtained at the reference hospitalization
Roentgenograms of the lumbar spine obtained at the follow-up examination
Radiographic evaluations and clinical material obtained from the record review
Forms FUA 10a and 10b for recording the results of the radiographic review (attached)
Instructions for completing these forms

Upon completion of the review, all materials were returned to the FUA for coding. A small sample of cases was used in a duplicate review to evaluate the reliability of these procedures.

VA COOPERATIVE STUDY OF THE NATURAL HISTORY OF LUMBAR DISC LESIONS

11 March 1964

Instructions for use of Form FUA R-20—10a and 10b for the review of radiologic materials

Forms 10a and 10b provide a means of recording the radiologic findings for the patients in this study on whom a follow-up examination has been performed. Three kinds of materials are to be reviewed:
1. Films taken at follow-up
2. Films taken during the reference hospitalization
3. Myelograms taken during the reference hospitalization

Included with the Army films will be copies of the Army x-ray reports obtained from the medical records of the veteran.

Continued.

Instructions for use of Forms FUA R20–10a and 10b—cont'd

Each case included in the review should have AP, lateral, and oblique views of the lumbosacral area taken during the follow-up examination. For patients who had fusion performed, three additional bending x-ray films should have been taken at follow-up showing the spine in extension, flexion, and lateral bending. Some cases will not have any x-ray films from the reference hospitalization period. Many will not have a myelogram.

One form 10a is to be filled out for each case with one or more myelogram films taken during the reference period. The form is required even if the myelogram shows no positive findings. A form 10a will not be included for cases without any myelogram films.

One form 10b is to be filled out to record any *positive findings* on the Army x-ray films taken during the reference period. In item A it should be indicated that the sheet summarizes positive findings on all the Army x-ray films taken during the reference hospitalization. Generally, cases with x-ray films or myelograms taken at reference hospitalization will also have follow-up x-ray films available. If the follow-up x-ray films show no abnormality, the part of item A "VA x-rays—Normal" should be circled when reviewing the Army x-ray films. Positive findings on the follow-up films should be recorded on a separate sheet. In rare instances there may be no follow-up films, and our staff will indicate this by marking the entry "No VA films available" on the 10b form supplied with the Army x-ray films.

One form 10b is to be filled out to record any *positive findings* on the x-ray films of the spine taken at the follow-up examination. In item A it should be indicated that the sheet summarizes all the x-ray films taken at VA follow-up. If there are no Army x-ray films from the reference period, our staff will indicate this by circling "No Army films available" on the sheet supplied with the VA follow-up films. If the Army films are available but show no positive findings, please indicate this by marking "Army x-rays—Normal" on the sheet used for the review of the VA follow-up films. If both the Army and the follow-up films are negative or missing, mark the appropriate combination in item A on one copy of form 10b and disregard the rest of the form.

Our staff will record the veteran's full name and case number on the sheet. Please be sure to check that you are reviewing the same case as that identified on the sheet. For cases with myelograms or any abnormal x-ray findings, all items on the appropriate form should be completed by circling one of the numbers provided for this purpose. If you find that an item of information cannot be determined from the x-ray materials for a given case, please indicate so by writing a note to that effect in the appropriate space on the form.

The following are instructions for several individual items on the form:

B, 3. When in doubt between "mild" and "moderate," or between "moderate" and "severe," use "moderate."

B, 4. Similarly, the identity of a transitional vertebra will be recorded as that identity most probably correct from evidence on available films. Include extranumerary or lumbarized S1 vertebrae.

B, 7. "Zero" in this space means that both right and left articulations at L5-S1 (or whatever numbers represent the lumbosacral junction) are sagittal. "One" means that the joint on the right deviates from the sagittal. "Two" means that the joint on the left deviates from sagittal. Indicate under "other" if asymmetry occurs at a higher level.

D, 1. Two opposing Schmorl's nodes will get two circles in the first column and one circle in the second column.

D, 3. "1" means congenital narrowing of more than average degree.

E   This section refers to acquired disc changes. Additional listings may have to be added if six lumbar vertebrae have been diagnosed.

E, 5. The term "fringing" is used to include "lipping" and "spurring."

M   Record definite evidence of specified or other relevant conditions. Item contains an abbreviation for calcification of the abdominal aorta.

Form FUA R20–10a

National Academy of Sciences–National Research Council
Follow-up Agency
R-20 Natural History of Lumbar Disc Lesions
Page 1 - Myelogram Films

NAS–NRC
FUA R20–10a Rev.
Dec. 1962

Case Number _____   Reviewer _____

Name _____   Date of Review _____

O   NO MYELOGRAM AVAILABLE (OMIT REST OF SHEET)

I   PRE-OPERATIVE MYELOGRAM (CIRCLE APPROPRIATE ITEMS EACH SPACE)   DATE OF FILM _____

A. Contrast Medium

1. Type	2. Amount Injected	3. Amount Aspirated	B. Technique 1. Level of Puncture	2. Needle Defect	3. Extent of Film Coverage	4. Adequate Views
1 Pantopaque	1 Less than 3cc	0 None	1 L1 – L2	0 Absent	1 Up to lower thoracic	1 P. A.
2 Lipiodol	2 3 – less than 6cc	1 All	2 L2 – L3	Present	2 Up to upper lumbar	2 Obliques
3 Air or O$_2$	3 6 – less than 9cc	2 ____ cc left (est. amount)	3 L3 – L4	1 Small	3 Up to mid lumbar	3 Prone lateral
4 Other –	4 9cc or more	3 Air myelogram	4 L4 – L5	2 Medium	4 Lower lumbar only	
V Unknown	V Unknown		5 L5 – S1	3 Large		
			V Unknown			

C. Interpretation

5. Complications	1. General	2. Anatomic Variations, Subarachnoid Space			3. Ligamentum Flavum Defect
		a. Congenitally Narrow Space	b. Congenitally Short Space	c. Unusually Wide Space	
0 None	0 Normal				0 No
1 Subdural, partial		0 No	0 No	0 No	
2 Subdural, complete	1 Abnormal				1 Yes
3 Extradural, partial		1 Yes	1 Yes	1 Yes	
4 Extradural, complete	2 Equivocal				
5 Intracranial oil					

4. Central Disc Protrusions			5. Posterolateral Protrusions		
a. Level	b. Defect in Oil Column	c. Nerve Roots	a. Level		b. Defect in Oil Column
0 No central protrusion (omit next 2 columns)	1 Complete obstruction	0 Normal	0 No posterolateral protrusion (omit next 2 columns)		1 Large
1 L1 – L2	2 Large, partial obstruction	1 Swollen	Right	Left	2 Moderate
2 L2 – L3			1 L1 – L2	1 L1 – L2	
3 L3 – L4	3 Moderate		2 L2 – L3	2 L2 – L3	3 Small
4 L4 – L5			3 L3 – L4	3 L3 – L4	
5 L5 – S1	4 Small		4 L4 – L5	4 L4 – L5	
			5 L5 – S1	5 L5 – S1	

c. Significant Minimal Deformities	6. Other Lesions	7. Estimation of Myelogram for Interpretation	II POST-OPERATIVE MYELOGRAM
	0 None		0 Not done or not available
0 None	1 Perineural cysts	1 Adequate	Post-operative adhesions
1 Loss of normal convexity of anterolateral margin	2 Lumbar or sacral meningoceles	2 Inadequate	1 Severe
2 Swollen nerve root	3 Angioma	Considerations for adequacy (Circle yes or no for each point)	2 Moderate
3 Displacement of oil col. (increased pedicle to oil distance)	4 Arachnoiditis		3 Mild
Nerve root sleeve	5 Tumor	Subarachnoid injection of contrast medium — Yes No	4 New protrusion at another level (specify)
4 Non filling	6 Other –	Proper level of puncture — Yes No	
5 Deformed		Adequate volume — Yes No	5 Oil column defect indicating recurrence at original site
6 Displaced		Adequate coverage — Yes No	
		Adequate views - P.A., obliques & prone lateral — Yes No	V Unable to satisfactorily interpret
		Significant anatomic variations — Yes No	

Continued.

Form FUA R20–10b

National Academy of Sciences–National Research Council

Case Number _____   Name _____

CIRCLE APPROPRIATE ITEMS IN EACH SPACE.
USE SEPARATE SHEETS IF BOTH ARMY AND VA FILMS ARE BEING REVIEWED.

Follow-up Agency
R-20 Natural History of Lumbar Disc Lesions
Page 2 - Plain films of Lumbar Spine (Army and VA)

A. Films Reviewed This Sheet

Army X-rays

0 No army films available
1 Normal (omit rest of sheet)
2 Abnormal (fill in following items)

VA X-rays

3 No VA films available
4 Normal (omit rest of sheet)
5 Abnormal (fill in following items)

B. Congenital Abnormalities

1. Spina Bifida

0 No
1 L1
2 L2
3 L3
4 L4
5 L5
6 S1
7 S2
8 S3

2. Spondylolysis

0 None or slight

Frank:

1 L1
2 L2
3 L3
4 L4
5 L5
6 S1

(Include Pars Interarticularis)

3. Spondylolisthesis

0 No

Mild	Moderate	Severe
1 L1-L2	1 L1-L2	1 L1-L2
2 L2-L3	2 L2-L3	2 L2-L3
3 L3-L4	3 L3-L4	3 L3-L4
4 L4-L5	4 L4-L5	4 L4-L5
5 L5-S1	5 L5-S1	5 L5-S1

4. Transitional Vertebra

0 No

Sacralization, L5
1 Right, with pseudoarthrosis
2 Right, without pseudoarthrosis
3 Left, with pseudoarthrosis
4 Left, without pseudoarthrosis

Lumbarization, S1
5 Right, with pseudoarthrosis
6 Right, without pseudoarthrosis
7 Left, with pseudoarthrosis
8 Left, without pseudoarthrosis

D. Developmental Abnormalities

1. Schmorl's Nodes

0 None or minimal

Frank:

Body	Space
1 L1	1 L1-L2
2 L2	2 L2-L3
3 L3	3 L3-L4
4 L4	4 L4-L5
5 L5	5 L5-S1
6 S1	

2. Limbus Vertebra - Irregular Contour and/or Defects

0 No
1 L1
2 L2
3 L3
4 L4
5 L5
6 S1

3. Narrow Lumbo-sacral Disc Space

0 None or slight
1 Frank narrowing

E. Acquired Disc Changes

1. Unusual Widening of Disc Space

0 No
1 L1-L2
2 L2-L3
3 L3-L4
4 L4-L5
5 L5-S1

2. Unusual Narrowing of Disc Space

0 No

Mild	Moderate	Severe
1 L1-L2	1 L1-L2	1 L1-L2
2 L2-L3	2 L2-L3	2 L2-L3
3 L3-L4	3 L3-L4	3 L3-L4
4 L4-L5	4 L4-L5	4 L4-L5
5 L5-S1	5 L5-S1	5 L5-S1

G. Lumbar Arthritis

1. Of Articular Facets

0 None or slight

Frank:

Right	Left
1 L1-L2	1 L1-L2
2 L2-L3	2 L2-L3
3 L3-L4	3 L3-L4
4 L4-L5	4 L4-L5
5 L5-S1	5 L5-S1

2. Rheumatoid Arthritis or Ankylosing Spondylitis

0 No
1 Yes

3. Kissing Posterior Spinous Process

0 No

Simple	False Joint
1 L1-L2	1 L1-L2
2 L2-L3	2 L2-L3
3 L3-L4	3 L3-L4
4 L4-L5	4 L4-L5
5 L5-S1	5 L5-S1

H. Arthritic Changes Sacro-iliac Joint

0 No

Right
1 Mild
2 Moderate
3 Severe

Left
4 Mild
5 Moderate
6 Severe

I. Vertebral Fracture

0 No

Body	Other than body - Specify anatomic site
1 L1	1 L1
2 L2	2 L2
3 L3	3 L3
4 L4	4 L4
5 L5	5 L5
6 S1	6 S1

Reviewer _____

Date of Review _____

NAS-NRC
FUA R20-10b Rev.
January 1964

5. Block Vertebra - Rudimentary Disc	6. Congenitally Flat Pedicles		7. Other Congenital Abnormalities	C. Changes in Spinal Contour		
				1. Scoliosis	2. Lumbar Lordosis	3. Lumbo-sacral Angle
0 No	0 No		0 None or minimal	0 No	0 Normal or slight deviation only	Use goniometer
1 L1-L2	Right	Left	Frank:	Convex to right		
2 L2-L3	1 L1	1 L1	1 Asymmetry articular facets L5-S1 without reaction	1 Mild	1 Loss of normal (marked)	_____ degrees
3 L3-L4	2 L2	2 L2		2 Moderate		
4 L4-L5	3 L3	3 L3		3 Severe	2 Exaggerated (marked)	
5 L5-S1	4 L4	4 L4	2 Asymmetry articular facets L5-S1 with reaction	Convex to left		
	5 L5	5 L5	3 Other (specify)	4 Mild		
	6 S1	6 S1		5 Moderate		
				6 Severe		

3. Calcification of Disc	4. Gas in Disc - Vacuum Phenomenon	5. Bony Fringing					6. Sclerosis of Adjacent Vertebral Surfaces		F. Neoplasm
0 None or slight	0 No	0 None or slight					0 None or slight		0 None
Frank calcification:	1 L1-L2	Frank:					Frank:		1 Present (spec. level and type)
Central	Posterior	2 L2-L3	Anterior	Posterior	Lateral		Body	Space	
					Right	Left			
1 L1-L2	1 L1-L2	3 L3-L4	1 L1-L2	1 L1-L2	1 L1-L2	1 L1-L2	1 L1	1 L1-L2	
2 L2-L3	2 L2-L3	4 L4-L5	2 L2-L3	2 L2-L3	2 L2-L3	2 L2-L3	2 L2	2 L2-L3	
3 L3-L4	3 L3-L4	5 L5-S1	3 L3-L4	3 L3-L4	3 L3-L4	3 L3-L4	3 L3	3 L3-L4	
4 L4-L5	4 L4-L5		4 L4-L5	4 L4-L5	4 L4-L5	4 L4-L5	4 L4	4 L4-L5	
5 L5-S1	5 L5-S1		5 L5-S1	5 L5-S1	5 L5-S1	5 L5-S1	5 L5	5 L5-S1	
							6 S1		

J. Inflammatory Process	K. Contrast Medium in Subarachnoid Space	L. Vertebral Fusion			M. Other Findings
		1. Type	2. Extent	3. Spinal Movement	
0 No	0 No	0 No fusion (omit next 2 columns)	Specify levels -	Flexion and Extension	0 None or possible Definite:
1 L1-L2	Yes	1 Bone		0 None or minimal	1 Hemangioma 2 Paget's disease
2 L2-L3	1 Diffuse	2 Metal		1 Significant movement	3 Fibrous dysplasia 4 Gen. osteoporosis
3 L3-L4	2 Localized (spec. level)	3 Bone and metal		Lateral bending	5 Previous Scheuermann's dis.
4 L4-L5		4 Other (spec.)		2 None or minimal,rt.	6 Sickle cell anemia
5 L5-S1	_____ cc (estimated amount)			3 Significant movement, right	7 Evidence of lamina removed (spec. level and side)
				4 None or minimal,lt.	8 Other (specify)
				5 Significant movement, left	

VARIABLES USED IN THE FACTOR ANALYSIS OF FOLLOW-UP
INFORMATION TO DEVELOP A SCORING OF DISABILITY

The methods used in obtaining and processing the observations are described in this Appendix. Each variable was scored so that the higher values indicate more disability. Unreported observations were assigned scores arbitrarily, usually the most frequently occurring score. The number of patients assigned each value of the score is given after the description of the scored item.

Observations on objective signs and events

1. *Atrophy of muscles of the legs*

   The circumference of the thigh and calf was measured. Differences of less than 1 cm. were not regarded as indicating atrophy.

Scoring	No. patients
0—No atrophy	327
0—Unknown status	3
1—Atrophy	459

2. *Weakness or spasm of muscles of the legs*

   This item summarizes the observation of mild, moderate, or severe weakness, or of visible contraction made on one or more of the following muscles: dorsal and plantar extensors of the foot, extensor hallucis longus, quadriceps femoris, and gluteal muscles.

Scoring	No. patients
0—No weakness	507
0—Unknown status	3
1—Weakness	279

3. *Decreased sensation in the legs*

   This information was coded by the physician in terms of the affected dermatome, or the affected area was represented in a drawing. Frequently both sources were available. A detailed evaluation of these responses in relation to each other and to the diagnosed level of lesion has been made elsewhere in this report.

Scoring	No. patients
0—No decreased sensation	382
0—Unknown status	41
1—Decreased sensation	366

4. *Decreased or absent reflexes of knee or ankle*

   Decreased or absent tendon reflexes of either knee or ankle were considered positive.

Scoring	No. patients
0—No decreased or absent reflexes	253
0—Unknown status	1
1—Decreased or absent reflexes	535

5. *Loss of lumbar lordosis*

   Observed at follow-up examination by the physician.

Scoring	No. patients
0—No loss of lordosis	544
0—Unknown status	8
1—Loss of lordosis	237

6. *Restriction of motion of lumbar spine*

The degrees of maximum forward flexion, extension, lateral bending, and rotation were recorded. Restriction was defined in the following ranges: flexion—0 to 69 degrees; extension—0 to 19 degrees; lateral bending—0 to 19 degrees; rotation—0 to 29 degrees.

Scoring	No. patients
0—No restriction in any direction	100
1—Flexion only restricted	28
1—Extension only restricted	40
1—Lateral bending or rotation or both restricted, without other restriction	157
1—Extension with lateral bending or rotation or both restricted, but no restriction of flexion	120
1—Unknown status	41
2—Flexion with other restriction	303

7. *Straight leg raising (SLR) test*

The maximum degrees of attainable leg raising were recorded.

Scoring	No. patients
0—Over 70 degrees in both legs or one leg unknown and the other 70 degrees+	477
0—Unknown status	10
1—70 degrees or less	302

8. *Changes in occupation determined from occupational history and work status*

The degree of change in occupation at entry into service, after discharge from service, and at the time of the follow-up examination is summarized in this item.

Scoring	No. patients
0—No change in occupation preservice to follow-up	174
1—Change preservice to follow-up	532
1—Unknown status	21
2—Not working now	62

Physician's evaluation of limitation and disability

9. *Limitation in use of back due to pain*

The physician evaluated whether use of back was limited by pain.

Scoring	No. patients
0—No limitation	242
1—Limitation	540
1—Unknown status	7

10. *Limitation in use of back due to weakness*

The physician evaluated whether use of back was limited by weakness.

Scoring	No. patients
0—No limitation	612
0—Unknown status	7
1—Limitation	170

11. *Limitation in use of legs*

The physician evaluated extent of limitation in running or walking.

Scoring	No. patients
0—No limitation	373
0—Unknown status	5
1—Limited running	303
2—Limited walking	108

12. *Degree of handicap in employment*

The physician evaluated degree of handicap in employment.

Scoring	No. patients
0—No handicap apparent	242
1—Some handicap	474
1—Unknown status	6
2—Severe handicap or unemployable	67

13. *Examiner's overall functional impression*

The physician evaluated patient's overall disability using a percent rating.

Scoring	No. patients
0—No disability due to disc	149
1—1% to 10%	298
1—Unknown status	28
2—11% to 20%	187
3—21% to 99%	127

Patient's evaluation of pain and disability

14. *Back pain*

The patient gave subjective report of extent of back pain.

Scoring	No. patients
0—None	104
1—Mild	305
1—Unknown status	7
2—Moderate	259
3—Severe	114

15. *Sciatica or leg pain*

The patient gave subjective report of extent of leg pain or sciatica.

Scoring	No. patients
0—None	297
0—Unknown status	7
1—Mild	247
2—Moderate	166
3—Severe	72

16. *Change in occupation due to disc disability*

The patient reported changes in employment due to disc disability.

Scoring	No. patients
0—No change, employed now, unemployed but not because of disc, changed jobs but not because of disc	409
0—Unknown status	5
1—Changed jobs or unemployed because of disc	375

Other information

17. *VA compensation rating for HNP disability as of June 1961, determined from VA claims folders*

Scoring	No. patients
0—Claim not filed, disallowed	79
1—Compensated 10%-29%	501
2—Compensated 30+% or retired for disability	209

18. *Surgery for HNP in the follow-up period to June 1961*

The VA claims folders were searched for evidence of VA or private hospitalizations, and the patients were questioned regarding interim surgery at the time of the examination.

Scoring	No. patients
0—No surgery for HNP	656
0—Unknown status	3
1—Surgery for HNP	130

SELECTED BIBLIOGRAPHY
1945-1970

Abbott, K. H., and Retter, R. H.: Antero-
lateral cordotomy for intractable pain
following unsuccessful disc surgery; a
review of fourteen cases, Bull. Los Angeles
Neurol. Soc. 23:112-118, 1958.

Abel, M. S.: Roentgenographic aspects of
post-traumatic arthritis, instability, and
disk deterioration following occult fractures of cervical spine, Clin. Orthop.
24:49-60, 1962.

Abel, M. S., and Harmon, P. H.: Oblique
motion studies and other non-myelo-
graphic roentgenographic criteria for diagnosis of traumatized or degenerated lumbar
intervertebral discs, Amer. J. Surg. 99:717-
729, 1960.

Adams, J. C.: Prolapsed intervertebral disc
with special reference to use and limitations of conservative treatment, Med.
Press 223:543-547, 1950.

Adams, J. C.: Intervertebral disc lesions and
their management, Med. Illus. 6:437-442,
1952.

Adams, J. E., and Inman, V. T.: Stretching
of the sciatic nerve; a means of relieving
postoperative pain following removal of
ruptured lumbar intervertebral discs, Calif.
Med. 91:24-26, 1959.

Aguilar, J. A., and Elvidge, A. R.: Intervertebral disk disease caused by the
Brucella organism, J. Neurosurg. 18:27-33,
1961.

Aho, A. J., Auranen, A., and Pesonen, K.:
Analysis of cauda equina symptoms in
patients with lumbar disc prolapse. Pre-
operative and follow-up clinical and cysto-
metric studies, Acta Chir. Scand. 135:413-
420, 1969.

Aitken, A. P.: Rupture of intervertebral disc
in industry; further observations on end
results, Amer. J. Surg. 84:261-267, 1952.

Aitken, A. P., and Bradford, C. H.: End
results of ruptured intervertebral discs in
industry, Amer. J. Surg. 73:365-380, 1947.

Albert, S. M., Rechtman, A. M., and
Kremens, V.: Significance of spinal fluid
protein level in intervertebral disk pathology, Penn. Med. 58:1235-1236, 1955.

Aldes, J. H., and Grabin, S.: Ultrasound in
the treatment of intervertebral disc syndrome, Amer. J. Phys. Med. 37:199-202
1958.

Aldes, J. H., and Koerner, F.: Rehabilitation
following ruptured intervertebral disc surgery, Arch. Phys. Med. 33:721-727, 1952.

Alexander, G. L.: Prolapsed intervertebral
disc, Edinburgh Med. J. 54:14-29, 1947.

Alfred, K. S.: Surgical treatment of herniated discs; follow-up study of 130 patients
without spinal fusion, Amer. J. Surg.
81:390-400, 1951.

Alpers, B. J.: Sciatica problem, Canad. Med.
Ass. J. 67:131-143, 1952.

Alpers, B. J.: Symposium on nervous and
mental diseases; neurological aspects of
sciatica, Med. Clin. N. Amer. 37:503-510,
1953.

Alvik, I.: Lumbar disc degeneration, Nord.
Med. 44:1318-1321, 1950.

Amsler, F. R., Jr., and Wilber, M. C.: Intra-
osseous vertebral venography as a diagnostic aid in evaluating intervertebral-disc
disease of the lumbar spine, J. Bone Joint
Surg. 49:703-712, 1967.

Anderson, H., and Roos, B. E.: Prognosis of
operatively treated lumbar disc herniations
causing foot extensor paralysis, Acta Chir.
Scand. 132:501-506, 1966.

Anderson, K. S., et al.: Comparative study
of myelographic filling defects in root
sheaths and operative findings in cases
of suspected lumbar intervertebral disc
herniation, Acta Orthop. Scand. 39:312-
320, 1968.

Anderson, T. P., Sachs, E., Jr., Fisher, R. G.,
and Krout, R. M.: Postoperative care in
lumbar disc syndrome, Arch. Phys. Med.
42:152-158, 1961.

Andrew, J.: Sacralization: aetiological factor
in lumbar intervertebral disk lesions, and
cause of misleading focal signs, Brit. J.
Surg. 42:304-311, 1954.

Arbuckle, R. K., Shelden, C. H., and
Pudenz, R. H.: Pantopaque myelography;
correlation of roentgenologic and neurologic findings, Radiology 45:356-369, 1945.

Arismendi, L.: Ruptured intervertebral disk,
Stanford Med. Bull. 5:68-70, 1947.

Arminio, J. A.: Trauma and the lumbar disc

lesion, Post-traumatic sequelae, Delaware Med. J. **39:**198-204, 1967.

Armstrong, J. R.: Causes of unsatisfactory results from operative treatment of lumbar disc lesions, J. Bone Joint Surg. **33-B:**31-35, 1951.

Armstrong, J. R.: Lumbar disc lesion syndrome, Rheumatism **9:**82-86, 1953.

Armstrong, J. R.: Lumbar disc lesions, Physiotherapy **50:**284-288, 1964.

Armstrong, J. R.: Lumbar disc lesions; pathogenesis and treatment of low back pain and sciatica, Edinburgh, 1965, E. & S. Livingstone, Ltd.

Armstrong, J. R.: The clinical picture in lumbar disc lesions, Brit. J. Clin. Pract. **20:**227-231, 1966.

Arnold, J. G., Jr.: "Sign of interlaminal tenderness," important aid in diagnosis and localization of intervertebral disc protrusions, Bull. Sch. Med. Univ. Maryland **35:**145-147, 1950.

Arnold, J. G., Jr.: End-results of surgery for protruded lumbar intervertebral discs; follow-up study of 364 cases over 6 and ½ year period, Bull. Sch. Med. Univ. Maryland **37:**3-8, 1952.

Aronson, H. A., and Dunsmore, R. H.: Herniated upper lumbar discs, J. Bone Joint Surg. **45-A:**311-317, 1963.

Arseni, C.: Clinical and statistical considerations on 5021 cases of hernia of lumbar discs, Rum. Med. Rev. **1:**55-57, 1957.

Arseni, C., and Nash, F.: Protrusion of thoracic intervertebral discs, Acta Neurochir. **11:**3-33, 1963.

Auld, A. W., Perlmutter, I., and Dooley, D. M.: Normal leg raising tests with herniated lumbar disk, J.A.M.A. **207:**2104, 1969.

Auld, A. W., Perlmutter, I., and Dooley, D. M.: Use of urea in the herniated intervertebral disc syndrome; a preliminary report, J. Florida Med. Ass. **56:**181-183. 1969.

Badgley, C. E.: Herniated disc; differential diagnosis and treatment, Chicago Med. Soc. Bull. **53:**399-406, 1950.

Bailey, F. W.: Decompression of the fifth lumbar nerve and intervertebral body fusions for low back pain with sciatic radiation, J. Int. Coll. Surg. **27:**160-169, 1957.

Bailey, R. W.: Observations of cervical intervertebral-disc lesions in fractures and dislocations, J. Bone Joint Surg. **45-A:**461-470, 1963.

Baker, A. H.: Lesion of intervertebral disk caused by lumbar puncture, Brit. J. Surg. **34:**385-388, 1947.

Bakhsh, A.: Ruptured intervertebral disc, Antiseptic **45:**464-466, 1948.

Bankart, A. S. B.: Low back pain and sciatica, Practitioner **157:**367-371, 1946.

Barbor, R.: Spinal traction, Lancet **1:**437-439, 1954.

Barbour, J. R.: Sciatica and such conditions of back as accompany it, Med. J. Aust. **1:**285-291, 1952.

Baro, W. Z.: Industrial intervertebral disk syndrome and its treatment as seen from psychiatric and neurologic viewpoint, Ann. Western Med. Surg. **5:**941-944, 1951.

Barr, J. S.: Ruptured intervertebral disc and sciatic pain, J. Bone Joint Surg. **29:**429-437, 1947.

Barr, J. S., and Craig, W. M.: Ruptured intervertebral disk, J. Nerv. Ment. Dis. **103:**688-701, 1946.

Barr, J. S., Kubik, C. S., and Molloy, M. K.: Evaluation of end results in treatment of ruptured lumbar intervertebral discs with protrusion of nucleus pulposus, Surg. Gynec. Obstet. **123:**250-256, 1967.

Barr, J. S., and Riseborough, E. J.: Treatment of low back and sciatic pain in patients over 60 years of age. A study of 100 patients, Clin. Orthop. **26:**12-18, 1963.

Barrada, Y., et al.: Neurologic complications of compression fracture of first lumbar vertebra, J. Roy. Egypt. Med. Ass. **34:**177-201, 1951.

Bartelink, D. L.: Myelography in intervertebral disk protrusion; horizontal beam examination with patient prone, Radiology **50:**202-206, 1948.

Batch, J. W., and Ashby, J. D.: Unusual cause of backache, U. S. Armed Forces Med. J. **7:**105-110, 1956.

Bauer, D.: Lumbar discography and low back pain, Springfield, Ill., 1960, Charles C Thomas, Publisher.

Begg, A. C.: Nuclear herniations of intervertebral disc; their radiological manifestations and significance, J. Bone Joint Surg. **36-B:**180-193, 1954.

Begg, A. C., and Falconer, M. A.: Plain radiography in intraspinal protrusion of lumbar intervertebral disks; correlation with operative findings, Brit. J. Surg. **36:**225-239, 1949.

Begg, A. C., Falconer, M. A., and McGeorge, M.: Myelography in lumbar intervertebral disk lesions; correlation with operative findings, Brit. J. Surg. **34:**141-157, 1946.

Bender, J. T., Jr.: Mechanical basis of low back pain, Alabama J. Med. Sci. **24:**217-218, 1955.

Berens, S. N.: Ruptured intervertebral disc syndrome. Is it an orthopedic or neurosurgical problem? J. Omaha Mid-West Clin. Soc. **7:**63-69, 1946.

Berg, A.: Clinical and myelographic studies of conservatively treated cases of lumbar intervertebral disc protrusion, Acta Chir. Scand. **104:**124-129, 1952.

Bettmann, E. H., and Neudorfer, R. J.: Cervical disk pathology resulting in dysphasia in an adolescent boy, New York J. Med. 60:2465-2467, 1960.

Black, H. A.: Massive herniation of intervertebral disc producing compression of cauda equina, Calif. Med. 69:271-274, 1948.

Blakey, P. R., Happey, F., Naylor, A., and Turner, R. L.: Protein in the nucleus pulposus of the intervertebral disk, Nature 195:73, 1962.

Blanche, D. W.: Ruptured intervertebral disc, Ann. Western Med. Surg. 4:240-244, 1950.

Blaschke, J. A.: Conservative management of intervertebral disc injuries, J. Okla. Med. Ass. 54:494-501, 1961.

Blau, J. N., and Logue, V.: Intermittent claudication of the cauda equina. An unusual syndrome resulting from central protrusion of a lumbar intervertebral disc, Lancet 1:1081-1086, 1961.

Blikra, G.: Intradural herniated lumbar disc, J. Neurosurg. 31:676-679, 1969.

Borak, J.: Spondylosis and spondylarthritis, Ann. Intern. Med. 26:427-439, 1947.

Borman, R. H.: Lumbosacral zygapophyseal tropism and the radiculodisk syndrome, J. Amer. Osteopath. Ass. 58:755-759, 1959.

Borski, A. A., and Smith, R. A.: Ureteral injury in lumbar-disc operation, J. Neurosurg. 17:925-928, 1960.

Boshes, L. D., and Lewin, P.: Guillain-Barré syndrome simulating herniated intervertebral disk, Illinois Med. J. 108:190-191, 1955.

Boult, G. F., Kiernan, M. K., and Childe, A. E.: Importance of minor myelographic deformities in diagnosis of posterior protrusion of lumbar vertebral disc, Amer. J. Roentgen. 66:752-763, 1951.

Boyd-Wilson, J. S.: Observations on the diagnosis of lumbar disc degeneration, New Zeal. Med. J. 60:202-206, 1961.

Boyle, A. C.: Role of the disc in backache, J. Roy. Inst. Public Health 21:123-132, 1958.

Bradford, D. S., and Garcia, A.: Herniations of the lumbar intervertebral disk in children and adolescents. A review of 30 surgically treated cases, J.A.M.A. 210:2045-2051, 1969.

Bradford, F. K.: Intervertebral disc rupture; appraisal of important signs, Dis. Nerv. Syst. 9:154-156, 1948.

Bradford, F. K.: Lumbar intervertebral disc rupture, Dis. Nerv. Syst. 11:3-19, 1950.

Bradford, F. K.: Low back and sciatic pain, J. Indiana Med. Ass. 50:559-563, 1957.

Bradford, F. K.: Lumbar intervertebral disc rupture: diagnosis, surgical treatment and complications, Amer. Surg. 24:908-918, 1958.

Bradford, F. K.: Low back sprain and ruptured intervertebral disc, Med. Times 00:707-808, 1960.

Bradford, F. K.: Ruptured intervertebral disk in the industrial patient: diagnosis, surgical management, and prognosis, Texas Med. 56:274-277, 1960.

Bradford, F. K.: Judgment in the management of low back and sciatic problems, Dis. Nerv. Syst. 22:520-524, 1961.

Bragdon, F. H., and Shafer, W. A.: Herniation of lumbar intervertebral disk; 10-year follow-up study, Penn. Med. 54:350-351, 1951.

Bragg, E. C., and Woodcock, J.: End result study of spine fusion for lumbosacral disorders excluding disk herniations, New York J. Med. 55:83-87, 1955.

Brailsford, J. F.: Lesions of intervertebral discs; some personal reflections, Brit. J. Radiol. 28:415-431, 1955.

Brain, R.: Heberdon oration, 1953: spondylosis; known and unknown, Ann. Rheum. Dis. 13:2-14, 1954; Lancet 1:687-693, 1954.

Brav, E. A., Molter, H. A., and Newcomb, W. J.: Lumbosacral articulation; roentgenologic and clinical study with special reference to narrow disc and lower lumbar displacement, Surg. Gynec. Obstet. 87:549-560, 1948.

Brendstrup, P., Jespersen, K., and Asboe-Hansen, G.: Morphological and chemical connective tissue changes in fibrositic muscles, Ann. Rheum. Dis. 16:438-440, 1957.

Breneman, J. C.: An original treatment method for the so-called herniated disc syndrome: clinical results and rationale, Curr. Ther. Res. 4:345-352, 1962.

Breneman, J. C.: The herniated disc syndrome. A logical sequence for examination and treatment, J. Occup. Med. 11:475-479, 1969.

Briggs, H., and Keats, S.: Clinical experiences in treatment of low back and sciatic pain associated with disorders of intervertebral discs, J. Med. Soc. New Jersey 43:13-18, 1946.

Briggs, H., and Keats, S.: Observations on obscure mechanisms of nerve-root compression with diagnostic tap test; report of 2 cases, J. Bone Joint Surg. 29:758-759, 1947.

Brodin, H.: Paths of nutrition in articular cartilage and intervertebral discs, Acta Orthop. Scand. 24:177-183, 1955.

Bromley, L. L., Craig, J. D., and Kessel, A. W. L.: Infected intervertebral disk after lumbar puncture, Brit. Med. J. 1:132-133, 1949.

Browder, J., and Watson, R.: Lesions of cervical intervertebral disc; clinicopathologic study of 22 cases, New York J. Med. **45:**730-737, 1945.

Browdie, A. S.: Evolution of surgery for intervertebral disc protrusion, Bull. Hosp. Joint Dis. **12:**75-79, 1951.

Brown, H. A., and Brown, B. A.: Lumbar intervertebral disk disease, Postgrad. Med. **37:**446-451, 1965.

Brown, H. A., and Pont, M. E.: Disease of lumbar discs. Ten years of surgical treatment, J. Neurosurg. **20:**410-417, 1963.

Brown, W. F., and Urie, G. N.: Herniated intervertebral disc, Treat. Serv. Bull. **8:**227-237, 1953.

Browne, K. M.: The role of diskography in the spectrographic analysis of the lumbar disk syndrome, Nebraska Med. J. **46:**99-104, 1961.

Buchstein, H. F.: Protruded intervertebral disc, J. Lancet **69:**264-270, 1949.

Bucy, P. C.: Neuroanatomical and neurosurgical aspects of herniated intervertebral discs, Instruct. Lect. Amer. Acad. Orthop. Surg. **18:**21-34, 1961.

Bucy, P. C., and Oberhill, H. R.: The diagnosis and treatment of herniated lumbar intervertebral discs, Chicago Med. **66:**201-205, 1963.

Burke, J. F., and Miller, J. W.: Chronaxie determinations in intervertebral disc pathology, J. Amer. Phys. Ther. Ass. **43:**265-267, 1963.

Burns, B. H., and Young, R. H.: Protrusion of intervertebral disc, Lancet **2:**424-427, 1945.

Burns, B. H., and Young, R. H.: Backache, Lancet **1:**623-626, 1947.

Burns, B. H., and Young, R. H.: Results of surgery in sciatica and low back pain, Lancet **1:**245-249, 1951.

Bush, H. D., Horton, W. G., Smare, D. L., and Naylor, A.: Fluid content of nucleus pulposus as factor in disk syndrome; further observations, Brit. Med. J. **2:**81-83, 1956.

Bush, L. F., and Engle, J. H.: Interbody fusions and the recurring disc problem, Bull. Geisinger Med. Cent. **14:**40-44, 1962.

Butterworth, R. D.: Spinal fusion in treatment of low back pain—some clinical observations, Virginia Med. Monthly **78:**551-553, 1951.

Caldwell, G. A., and Sheppard, W. B.: Criteria for spine fusion following removal of protruded nucleus pulposus, J. Bone Joint Surg. **30-A:**971-980, 1948.

Caldwell, G. A., and Sheppard, W. B.: Lumbosacral fusion vs. laminectomy for protrusion of IV disc for selected cases of low back pain with sciatic radiation, Mississippi Doctor **25:**379-380, 1948.

Cameron, B. M., and Holmes, T. W., Jr.: Acute infection of lumbar intervertebral disc treated by anterior resection and drainage; report of case, Southern Med. J. **48:**1190-1192, 1955.

Cameron, J. A. P.: Intervertebral disc in relation to low back pain, Med. J. Malaya **8:**28-44, 1953.

Camp, J. D.: Contrast myelography, Amer. Acad. Orthop. Surg. Lect. **12:**243-253, 1955.

Campbell, A. M., and Phillips, D. G.: Cervical disk lesions with neurological disorder. Differential diagnosis, treatment, and prognosis, Brit. Med. J. **2:**481-485, 1960.

Campbell, E., and Whitfield, R. D.: Certain reasons for failure following disk operations, New York Med. **47:**2569-2573, 1947.

Cannon, B. W., Hunter, S. E., and Picaza, J. A.: Nerve-root anomalies in lumbardisc surgery, J. Neurosurg. **19:**208-214, 1962.

Capener, N.: Clinical significance and treatment of lesions of intervertebral disk, Ann. Rheum. Dis. **8:**59-63, 1949.

Carpenter, E. B.: Methocarbamol as a muscle relaxant: its clinical evaluation in acute trauma and chronic neurological states, S. Dakota J. Med. **51:**627-630, 1958.

Case records of the Massachusetts General Hospital: Case 45402, New Eng. J. Med. **261:**715-720, 1959.

Chandler, F. A.: Herniated intervertebral disk, Industr. Med. Surg. **18:**283-287, 1949.

Chang, C. Y.: Studies on the intervertebral disk herniation at the lumbar spine (as a cause of sciatica and low back pain), J. Formosan Med. Ass. **62:**292-309, 1963.

Charlton, W. S.: Whither the disk? Med. J. Aust. **43:**857-858, 1956.

Charlton, W. S.: Review of the present position in spinal intervertebral disc disease, Med. J. Aust. **49:**581-586, 1962.

Charnley, J.: Orthopaedic signs in diagnosis of disc protrusion, with special reference to straight-leg-raising test, Lancet **1:**186-192, 1951.

Charnley, J.: Inhibition of fluid as cause of herniation of nucleus pulposus, Lancet **1:**124-127, 1952.

Clark, F. J.: Recent advances in surgical treatment of lumbar intervertebral disk disease, Med. J. Aust. **1:**49-52, 1946.

Clark, G. G.: Operative results in lumbar disk syndrome; majority of patients return to full duty, U. S. Armed Forces Med. J. **8:**195-197, 1957.

Cleveland, D.: Interspace reconstruction and spinal stabilization after disc removal, J. Lancet **76:**327-331, 1956.

Cloward, R. B.: Anterior herniation of ruptured lumbar intervertebral disk; comments on diagnostic value of diskogram, Arch. Surg. **64:**457-463, 1952.

Cloward, R. B.: Changes in vertebra caused

by ruptured intervertebral discs; observations on their formation and treatment, Amer. J. Surg. 84:151-161, 1952.

Cloward, R. B.: Lumbar intervertebral disc surgery; description of new instrument, vertebra spreader, Surgery 32:852-857, 1952.

Cloward, R. B.: Recent improvements in surgical treatment of low back pain due to ruptured lumbar intervertebral discs, Hawaii Med. J. 11:279-285, 1952.

Cloward, R. B.: Treatment of ruptured lumbar intervertebral disc by vertebral body fusion; method of use of banked bone, Ann. Surg. 136:987-992, 1952.

Cloward, R. B.: Treatment of ruptured lumbar intervertebral discs by vertebral body fusion; indications, operative technique, after care, J. Neurosurg. 10:154-168, 1953.

Cloward, R. B.: Treatment of ruptured lumbar intervertebral discs; criteria for spinal fusion, Amer. J. Surg. 86:145-151, 1953.

Cloward, R. B.: Degenerated lumbar disc: treatment by vertebral body fusion, J. Int. Coll. Surg. 22:375-386, 1954.

Cloward, R. B.: Multiple ruptured lumbar discs, Ann. Surg. 142:190-195, 1955.

Cloward, R. B.: Vertebral body fusion for ruptured lumbar discs; roentgenographic study, Amer. J. Surg. 90:969-976, 1955.

Cloward, R. B.: Vertebral body fusion for ruptured cervical discs, Amer. J. Surg. 98:722-727, 1959.

Cloward, R. B.: The clinical significance of the sinu-vertebral nerve of the cervical spine in relation to the cervical disk syndrome, J. Neurol. Neurosurg. Psychiat. 23:321-326, 1960.

Cloward, R. B.: New method of diagnosis and treatment of cervical disc disease, Clin. Neurosurg. 8:93-132, 1962.

Cloward, R. B.: Lesions of the intervertebral disks and their treatment by interbody fusion methods. The painful disk, Clin. Orthop. 27:51-77, 1963.

Cloward, R. B.: Surgical treatment of traumatic cervical spine syndrome, Wiederherstellungschir. Traum. 7:148-185, 1963.

Cloward, R. B., and Buzaid, L. L.: Discography; technique, indications and evaluation of normal and abnormal intervertebral disc, Amer. J. Roentgen. 68:552-564, 1952.

Code, C. F., Williams, M. M. D., Baldes, E. J., and Ghormley, R. K.: Are intervertebral disks displaced during positive acceleration? J. Aviat. Med. 18:231-236, 1947.

Cohen, R., Burnip, R., and Wagner, E.: Calcification of intervertebral disc in child; report of case study, Ann. Western Med. Surg. 3:202-204, 1949.

Cole, H. G., and Wilson, A. A.: An adjunct in office treatment of low back syndrome, J. Florida Med. Ass. 42:643-645, 1956.

Collis, J. S., Jr., and Gardner, W. J.: Lumbar discography. Analysis of 600 degenerated disks and diagnosis of degenerative disk disease, J.A.M.A. 178:67-70, 1961.

Collis, J. S., Jr., and Gardner, W. J.: Lumbar discography. An analysis of one thousand cases, J. Neurosurg. 19:452-461, 1962.

Colonna, P. C., and Friedenberg, Z. B.: Disc syndrome; results of conservative care of patients with positive myelograms, J. Bone Joint Surg. 31-A:614-618, 1949.

Compere, E. L.: Fusion of spine after removal of ruptured disk, J. Int. Coll. Surg. 9:14-19, 1946.

Compere, E. L.: Origin, anatomy, physiology, and pathology of the intervertebral disc, Instruct. Lect. Amer. Acad. Orthop. Surg. 18:15-20, 1961.

Congdon, C. C.: Proliferative lesions resembling chordoma following puncture of nucleus pulposus in rabbits, J. Nat. Cancer Inst. 12:893-907, 1952.

Coplans, C. W.: Lumbar disc herniation; effect of torque on its causation and conservative treatment; preliminary report, S. Afr. Med. J. 25:881-884, 1951.

Coplans, C. W.: Lumbar intervertebral disc herniation; method of conservative treatment, S. Afr. Med. J. 27:182-187, 1953.

Corboy, P. H.: Medical testimony in a lumbar intervertebral disc injury case, showing the direct and cross-examination of the neurosurgeon, Med. Trial. Techn. Quart. 9:73-123, 1962.

Coventry, M. B., Ghormley, R. K., and Kernohan, J. W.: Intervertebral disc; its microscopic anatomy and pathology; anatomy, development, and physiology, J. Bone Joint Surg. 27:105-112, 1945.

Coventry, M. B., Ghormley, R. K., and Kernohan, J. W.: Intervertebral disc; its microscopic anatomy and pathology; changes in intervertebral disc concomitant with age, J. Bone Joint Surg. 27:233-237, 1945.

Coventry, M. B., Ghormley, R. K., and Kernohan, J. W.: Intervertebral disc; its microscopic anatomy and pathological changes in intervertebral disc, J. Bone Joint Surg. 27:460-474, 1945.

Craig, W. M., Svien, H. J., Dodge, H. W., Jr., and Camp, J. D.: Intraspinal lesions masquerading as protruded lumbar intervertebral disks, J.A.M.A. 149:250-253, 1952.

Crisp, E. J.: Damaged intervertebral disk; early diagnosis and treatment, Lancet 2:422-424, 1945.

Crisp, E. J.: Treatment of lumbar disc lesions by immobilization in plaster jacket, Rheumatism 4:211-213, 1948.

Crisp, E. J., Kersley, G. D., and Kininmouth, D. A.: Discussion on manipulation, Ann. Phys. Med. 1:134-144, 1952.

Crawford, A. S.: Nerve compression syndrome of lumbar nerves, modern concepts and surgical treatment, J. Maine Med. Ass. **36**:183-187, 1945.

Crawford, A. S., Mitchell, C. L., and Granger, G. R.: Surgical treatment of low back pain with sciatica radiation; preliminary report of 346 cases, Arch. Surg. **59**:724-730, 1949.

Crock, H. V.: A reappraisal of intervertebral disc lesions, Med. J. Aust. **1**:983-989, 1970.

Cronquist, S.: The postoperative myelogram, Acta Radiol. **52**:45-51, 1959.

Crosett, A. D., Jr.: Calcification of intervertebral discs in child; report of case following poliomyelitis, J. Pediat. **47**:481-484, 1955.

Cyriax, J.: Lumbago; mechanism of dural pain, Lancet **2**:427-429, 1945.

Cyriax, J.: Treatment of lumbar disc lesions, Brit. Med. J. **2**:1434-1438, 1950.

Cyriax, J.: Treatment of lumbar disc-lesions, Postgrad. Med. **29**:4-10, 1953.

Cyriax, J.: Spinal disk lesions; assessment after 21 years, Brit. Med. J. **1**:140-142, 1955.

Cyriax, J.: Lumbar disc lesions; conservative treatment, S. Afr. Med. J. **32**:1-3, 1958.

Cyriax, J.: Conservative treatment of lumbar disc lesions, Physiotherapy **50**:300-303, 1964.

Cyriax, J.: Manipulation for lumbar disc prolapse, Brit. Med. J. **4**:173, 1969.

Dahlgren, S.: Results of early operative treatment of sciatica, Acta Orthop. Scand. **33**:18-23, 1963.

Dandy, W. E.: Treatment of spondylolisthesis, J.A.M.A. **127**:137-139, 1945.

Daniel, E. F., and Smith, G. W.: Foreignbody granuloma of intervertebral disc and spinal cord, J. Neurosurg. **17**:480-482, 1960.

Daum, H. F., Smith, A. B., Walker, J. W., Chapman, S. B., and Eversman, G. H.: Protrusions of the lumbar disk; a correlation of the radiographic diagnoses and surgical findings, Southern Med. J. **52**:1479-1484, 1959.

Davidson, E. A., and Woodhall, B.: Biochemical alterations in herniated intervertebral disks, J. Biol. Chem. **234**:2951-2954, 1959.

Davies, F. L.: Problems of lumbar intervertebral disc injuries and their importance in industry, Trans. Ass. Industr. Med. Off. **2**:84-87, 1952.

Davies, F. L.: Late results of lumbar intervertebral disc injuries in industry, Industr. Med. Surg. **24**:497-499, 1955.

Davies, J. J., and Peirce, E. C., II: Discography in diagnosis of herniation of lower lumbar intervertebral discs, Illinois Med. J. **104**:118-125, 1953.

Davis, A. G.: Symposium on intervertebral disc; introduction, J. Bone Joint Surg. **29**:424-425, 1947.

Davis, L., Martin, J., and Goldstein, S. L.: Sensory changes with herniated nucleus pulposus, J. Neurosurg. **9**:133-138, 1952.

Dawson, G. R., Jr.: A diagnostic sign in fourth and fifth lumbar disc surgery. The so-called jerk reflex, J. Bone Joint Surg. **51**:1660, 1969.

Day, P. L., and Hinchey, J. J.: Herniated intervertebral lumbar discs operated upon: a follow-up study of some 200 cases, Southern Med. J. **55**:663-666, 1962.

Decker, H. G.: Extensive paralysis from protruded intervertebral discs in the lumbar area; a report of two cases, J. Iowa Med. Soc. **47**:512-513, 1957.

Decker, H. G., and Brennan, J. E.: Review of 50 operated cases of protruded or ruptured intervertebral discs in lumbar areas, J. Iowa Med. Soc. **41**:215-218, 1951.

Decker, H. G., and Shapiro, S. W.: Herniated lumbar intervertebral disks; results of surgical treatment without the routine use of spinal fusion, Arch. Surg. **75**:77-84, 1957.

de Gispert-Cruz, I., and Escarpenter, G. J.: Compressive and neuritic sciatica, Rheumatism **10**:35-38, 1954.

Della Pietra, A.: Stabilizing spinal fusion following herniated disk removal without fusion, J.A.M.A. **157**:701-702, 1955.

DePalma, A. F., and Gillespy, T., Jr.: Longterm results of herniated nucleus pulposus treated by excision of the disc only, Clin. Orthop. **22**:139-144, 1962.

DePalma, A. F., and Rothman, R. H.: Surgery of the lumbar spine, Clin. Orthop. **63**:162-170, 1969.

Deutsch, I.: The use of simple roentgen methods in intervertebral disk syndrome diagnosis, J. Florida Med. Ass. **47**:523-526, 1960.

Deutsch, I.: Thoughts about intervertebral disks, Southern Med. J. **54**:50-53, 1961.

Dixon, F. W. P., and Kiernander, B.: Physiotherapy in treatment of prolapsed intervertebral discs, Brit. J. Phys. Med. **16**:221-223, 1953.

Donaghy, R. M. P.: Posterior tibial reflex; reflex of some value in localization of protruded intervertebral disc in lumbar region, J. Neurosurg. **3**:457-459, 1946.

Drechsler, B., et al.: Electrophysiological study of patients with herniated intervertebral discs, Electromyography **6**:187-204, 1966.

Duffy, J. J., Basile, J. X., and Voris, H. C.: Results of operations for lumbar disc protrusions, Amer. J. Surg. **100**:434-438, 1960.

Dunning, H. S.: Prognosis in so-called sciatic neuritis, Arch. Neurol. Psychiat. **55**:573-577, 1946.

du Toit, J. G.: Herniation of the nucleus pulposus in lumbar region, S. Afr. Med. J. 23:391-393, 1949.

Echlin, F. A., Ivie, J. M., and Fine, A.: Pantopaque myelography as aid in pre-operative diagnosis of protruded inter-vertebral discs; preliminary report, Surg. Gynec. Obstet. 80:257-260, 1945.

Echlin, F. A., Selverstone, B., and Scribner, W. E.: Bilateral and multiple ruptured discs as one cause of persistent symptoms following operation for herniated disc, Surg. Gynec. Obstet. 83:485-493, 1946.

Echols, D. H.: Surgical treatment of sciatica; results 3 to 8 years after operation, Arch. Neurol. Psychiat. 61:672-679, 1949.

Echols, D. H., and Rehfeldt, F. C.: Failure to disclose ruptured intervertebral disks in 32 operations for sciatica, J. Neurosurg. 6:376-382, 1949.

Ecker, A.: Kneeling position for operations on lumbar spine, especially for protruded intervertebral disc, Surgery 25:112, 1949.

Ecker, A.: Oblique variation of cross-table lateral (horizontal beam) myelography, J. Neurosurg. 19:264-265, 1962.

Eckert, C., and Decker, A.: Pathological studies of intervertebral discs, J. Bone Joint Surg. 29:447-454, 1947.

Eckhoff, N. L.: Disc lesion, Guy Hosp. Gaz. 64:4-10, 1950.

Edeiken, J., Wallace, J. D., and Curley, R. F., et al.: Thermography and herniated lumbar disks, Amer. J. Roentgen. 102:790-796, 1968.

Edgren, W., Heikel-Pursiainen, U., and Karaharju, E. O.: Herniation lumbar discs in one thousand myelograms, Ann. Chir. Gynaec. Fenn. 55:135-138, 1966.

Eie, N.: Combined extirpation and spinal fusion in lumbar intervertebral disk herni-ations. Follow-up examinations of 282 patients, J. Oslo City Hosp. 14:149-174, 1964.

Eie, N., and Kristiansen, K.: Complications and hazards of traction in the treatment of ruptured lumbar intervertebral disks, J. Oslo City Hosp. 12:5-12, 1962.

Ekengren, K., and Lindblom, K.: Dissecting disc herniation in a 4-year-old child, Acta Radiol. 48:156-158, 1957.

Emmett, J. L., and Love, J. G.: Urinary re-tention in women caused by asympto-matic protruded lumbar disk: report of 5 cases, J. Urol. 99:597-606, 1968.

English, R. H., and Spriggs, J. B.: Pain path-ways in herniated nucleus pulposus syn-drome; preliminary report, Milit. Surg. 102:213-216, 1948.

Epstein, B. S.: Low back pain associated with varices of epidural veins simulating herni-ation of nucleus pulposus, Amer. J. Roent-gen. 57:736-740, 1947.

Epstein, B. S.: Complete block of lumbar

spinal canal due to herniation of nucleus pulposus, Amer. J. Roentgen. 61:775-783, 1949.

Epstein, J. A., Epstein, B. S., and Lavine, L.: Nerve root compression associated with narrowing of the lumbar spinal canal, J. Neurol. Neurosurg. Psychiat. 25:165-176, 1962.

Epstein, J. A., and Lavine, L. S.: Herniated lumbar intervertebral discs in teen-age children, J. Neurosurg. 21:1070-1075, 1964.

Epstein, J. A., Lavine, L. S., Epstein, B. S., et al.: Herniated disks and related dis-orders of the lumbar spine. Surgical treat-ment in the geriatric patient, J.A.M.A. 202:187-190, 1967.

Epstein, J. A., Lavine, L. S., and Epstein, B. S.: Recurrent herniation of the lumbar intervertebral disk, Clin. Orthop. 52:169-178, 1967.

Erickson, T. C.: Syndrome of intervertebral disk, Wisconsin Med. J. 46:898-900, 1947.

Erlacher, P. R.: Nucleography, J. Bone Joint Surg. 34-B:204-210, 1952.

Eyre-Brook, A. L.: Study of late results from disk operations; present employment and residual complaints, Brit. J. Surg. 39:289-296, 1952.

Fahrenkung, A., Gottschalck, B., and Hoj-gaard, K.: Myelography with water-solu-able media in lumbago-sciatica after oper-ation for herniated lumbar disk, Acta Radiol. 2:138-144, 1964.

Fairburn, B., and Steward, J. M.: Lumbar disc protrusion as surgical emergency, Lancet 2:319-321, 1955.

Falconer, M. A., Glasgow, G. L., and Cole, D. S.: Sensory disturbances occurring in sciatica due to intervertebral disc protru-sions; some observations on fifth lumbar and first sacral dermatomes, J. Neurol. Neurosurg. Psychiat. 10:72-84, 1947.

Falconer, M. A., McGeorge, M., and Begg, A. C.: Surgery of lumbar intervertebral disc protrusion; study of principles and results based upon 100 consecutive cases submitted to operation, Brit. J. Surg. 35:225-249, 1948.

Feffer, H. L.: Treatment of low-back and sci-atic pain by injection of hydrocortisone into degenerated discs, J. Bone Joint Surg. 38-A:585-592, 1956.

Fernström, U.: Protruded lumbar interver-tebral disc in children; case report of a case and review of literature, Acta Chir. Scand. 111:71-79, 1956.

Fernström, U.: Lumbar intervertebral disc degeneration with abdominal pain, Acta Chir. Scand. 113:436-437, 1957.

Fernström, U.: A discographical study of rup-tured lumbar intervertebral discs, Acta Chir. Scand. supp. 258:1-60, 1960.

Fernström, U.: Anthroplasty with intercorporal endoprosthesis in herniated disc and in painful disc, Acta Chir. Scand. supp. 357:154+, 1966.

Fernström, U.: Ruptured lumbar discs causing abdominal pain, Acta Chir. Scand. supp. 357:160+, 1966.

Fernström, U., and Goldie, I.: Does granulation tissue in the intervertebral disc provoke low back pain? Acta Orthop. Scand. 30:202-206, 1960.

Ferry, A. M.: Degenerative disc syndrome of low back, Virginia Med. Monthly 83:146-150, 1956.

Fincher, E. F.: Differential diagnosis of intervertebral cartilage ruptures and intraspinal tumors within lumbar sacral canal, Southern Surg. 12:292-304, 1946.

Firtel, S. L.: Posterior central herniation of intervertebral disc diagnosed after lumbosacral and sacroiliac fusion, Bull. Hosp. Joint Dis. 7:154-160, 1946.

Fischer, A. G.: Manipulation in lumbar intervertebral disc lesions, Practitioner 187:319-328, 1961.

Fisher, R. G., and Williams, J.: Ochronosis associated with degeneration of intervertebral disc, J. Neurosurg. 12:403-406, 1955.

Flax, H. J., Berrios, R., and Rivera, D.: Electromyography in the diagnosis of herniated lumbar disc, Arch. Phys. Med. 45:520-524, 1964.

Flaxman, N.: Lumbar intervertebral disc syndromes, Med. Trial Techn. Quart. 9:37-71, 1961.

Fletcher, G. H.: Backward displacement of fifth lumber vertebra in degenerative disc disease; significance of difference in anteroposterior diameters of fifth lumber and first sacral vertebrae, J. Bone Joint Surg. 29:1019-1026, 1947.

Flinchum, D.: Closed treatment of herniated intervertebral lumbar discs, J. Med. Ass. Georgia 48:461-464, 1959.

Foltz, E. L., Ward, A. A., and Knopp, L. M.: Intervertebral fusion following lumbar disc excision, J. Neurosurg. 13:469-478, 1956.

Forbes, G.: An improvised perspex spinal splint, J. Roy. Nav. Med. Serv. 43:219-221, 1957.

Ford, L. T., and Key, J. A.: Evaluation of myelography in diagnosis of intervertebral-disc lesions in low back, J. Bone Joint Surg. 32-A:257-266,306, 1950.

Ford, L. T., and Key, J. A.: Experimental production of intervertebral disc lesions by chemical injury, Surg. Forum (1951), pp. 447-452, 1952.

Ford, L. T., and Key, J. A.: Postoperative infection of intervertebral disc space, Southern Med. J. 48:1295-1303, 1955.

Ford, L. T., Ramsey, R. H., Holt, E. P., and Key, J. A.: Analysis of 100 consecutive lumbar myelograms followed by disc operations for relief of low-back pain and sciatica, Surgery 32:961-966, 1952.

Fortune, C.: Arterio-venous fistula of left common iliac artery and vein, Med. J. Aust. 43:660-661, 1956.

Fraser, W. N.: The operative treatment of prolapsed discs in the lumbar region, New Zeal. Med. J. 65:437-443, 1966.

Fredrickson, D.: A physical therapy program for the postoperative herniated nucleus pulposus patient, Phys. Ther. Rev. 37:458-459, 1957.

Freeman, D. G.: Major vascular complications of lumbar disc surgery, Western J. Surg. 60:175-177, 1961.

Freeman, L. W.: Surgical treatment of back and leg pain persisting after adequate disc surgery, J. Indiana Med. Ass. 54:1265-1267, 1961.

Friberg, S.: Anatomical studies on lumbar disc degeneration, Acta Orthop. Scand. 17:224-230, 1948.

Friberg, S.: Lumbar disc degeneration in problem of lumbago sciatica (Sir Robert Jones lecture), Bull. Hosp. Joint Dis. 15:1-20, 1954.

Friberg, S., and Hirsch, C.: On late results of operative treatment for intervertebral disc prolapses in lumbar region; preliminary report, Acta Chir. Scand. 93:161-168, 1946.

Friberg, S., and Hirsch, C.: Anatomical and clinical studies on lumbar disc degeneration, Acta Orthop. Scand. 19:222-242, 1949.

Friberg, S., and Hult, L.: Comparative study of abrodil myelogram and operative findings in low back pain and sciatica, Acta Orthop. Scand. 20:303-314, 1951.

Friedenberg, Z. B.: Symposium on orthopedic surgery; results of nonoperative treatment of ruptured lumbar disks, Surg. Clin. N. Amer. 33:1545-1549, 1953.

Friedenberg, Z. B., Broder, H. A., Edeiken, J. E., and Spencer, H. N.: Degenerative disk disease of cervical spine. Clinical and roentgenographic study, J.A.M.A. 174:375-380, 1960.

Friedenberg, Z. B., and Shoemaker, R. C.: Results of non-operative treatment of ruptured lumbar discs, Amer. J. Surg. 88:933-935, 1954.

Friedman, H.: Intraspinal rheumatoid nodule causing nerve root compression; case report, J. Neurosurg. 32:689-691, 1970.

Friedman, J., and Goldner, M. Z.: Discography in evaluation of lumbar disk lesions, Radiology 65:653-662, 1955.

Fulcher, O. H.: Syndrome of the ruptured fourth dorsal intervertebral disc, Georgetown Med. Bull. 16:159-161, 1963.

Fulford, P. C.: Surgery for lumbar disc protrusions, J. Roy. Nav. Med. Serv. 56:92-97, 1970.

Gage, E. L., and Shafer, W. A.: Herniation of lumbar intervertebral disks in coal miners; preliminary report, Amer. Surg. 19:577-583, 1953.

Gama, C.: Neuralgic pain wrongly ascribed to posterior hernia of intervertebral discs; 2 cases, J. Int. Coll. Surg. 13:578-582, 1950.

Garceau, G. J.: Simple disc surgery versus combined operation, Southern Med. J. 44:213-216, 1951.

Gardner, R. C.: The lumbar intervertebral disk. A clinicopathological correlation based on over 100 laminectomies, Arch. Surg. 100:101-104, 1970.

Gardner, W. J., et al.: X-ray visualization of intervertebral disk with consideration of morbidity of disk puncture, Arch. Surg. 64:355-364, 1952.

Gates, E. M., and Morton, J. A.: Venous malformations of spinal meninges, Surg. Forum (1951), pp. 388-395, 1952.

Geiger, L. E.: Fusion of vertebrae following resection of intervertebral disc, J. Neurosurg. 18:79-85, 1961.

Genest, A. S.: Results of surgical treatment in 100 consecutive cases of lumbar herniated disc syndrome, Med. Bull. U. S. Army Europe 20:272-274, 1963.

Gershon-Cohen, J.: Phantom nucleus pulposus, Amer. J. Roentgen. 56:43-48, 1946.

Gershon-Cohen, J., Schraer, H., Sklaroff, D. M., and Blumberg, N.: Dissolution of intervertebral disk in the aged normal; phantom nucleus pulposus, Radiology 62:383-386, 1954.

Gillespie, H. W.: Radiologic diagnosis of lumbar intervertebral disc lesions; report on 160 cases, Brit. J. Radiol. 19:420-428, 1946.

Glass, B. A., and Ilgenfritz, H. C.: Arteriovenous fistula secondary to operation for ruptured intervertebral disc, Ann. Surg. 140:122-127, 1954.

Gleason, P. G.: Technique of discography, U. S. Armed Forces Med. J. 3:1831-1837, 1952.

Glorieux, P.: Considèrations au sujet du diagnostic de la hernie postèrieure du mènisque intervertèbral, Acta Radiol. 34:299-308, 1950.

Gol, A.: Treatment of disk lesions of the lumbar spine by intradisk injections of enzymes, Southern Med. J. 59:1293-1296, 1966.

Goldenberg, R.: Herniation of lumbar intervertebral disc, Bull. Hosp. Joint Dis. 9:117-123, 1948.

Goldenberg, R.: Diagnostic difficulties in herniated disk, J. Med. Soc. New Jersey 49:455-458, 1952.

Goldenberg, R.: Diagnostic problems in herniated intervertebral disc, Bull. Hosp. Joint Dis. 14:86-100, 1953.

Goldie, I.: Granulation tissue in the ruptured intervertebral disc, Acta Path. Microbiol. Scand. 42:302-304, 1958.

Goldner, J. L.: Lesions in the back and lower extremities which may simulate ruptured disk, N. Carolina Med. J. 17:260-267, 1956.

Gomibuchi, R.: Electron microscope studies on the fine structure of the intervertebral disc, with special reference to intervertebral disc herniation, J. Jap. Orthop. Ass. 37:1027-1041, 1964.

Gordon, E. E.: Natural history of the intervertebral disc, Arch. Phys. Med. 42:750-763, 1961.

Gottschalck, B., and Hojgaard, K.: Operatively treated patients with herniated lumbar disk, but without objective radicular findings, Acta Neurol. Scand. 38:261-265, 1962.

Gottschalck, B., and Hojgaard, K.: Operatively treated patients with lumbago-sciatica, without demonstrable herniation of the disk, Acta Neurol. Scand. 38:266-270, 1962.

Gottschalck, B., and Hojgaard, K.: Results of operation for herniated lumbar disk, Acta Neurol. Scand. 38:256-260, 1962.

Graf, C. J., and Hamby, W. B.: Roentgenographic demonstration by tantalum powder of sinuses resulting from extraction of intervertebral disc protrusions, Amer. J. Roentgen. 53:157-160, 1945.

Graf, C. J., and Hamby, W. B.: Paraplegia in lumbar intervertebral disk protrusions with remarks on high lumbar disk herniation, New York J. Med. 53:2346-2348, 1953.

Grant, F. C.: Operative results of intervertebral disks, Ann. Surg. 124:1066-1075, 1946.

Grant, F. C., Austin, G., Friedenberg, Z. B., and Hansen, A.: Correlation of neurologic, orthopedic, and roentgenographic findings in displaced intervertebral discs, Surg. Gynec. Obstet. 87:561-568, 1948.

Grant, F. C., and Nulsen, F. E.: Symposium on safeguards in surgical diagnosis: ruptured intervertebral discs, Surg. Clin. N. Amer. 32:1777-1790, 1952.

Grantham, E. G., and Spurling, R. G.: Symposium on nervous and mental diseases; ruptured lumbar intervertebral disks, Med. Clin. N. Amer. 37:479-502, 1953.

Grantham, S. A.: Herniated lumbar disc, Amer. J. Surg. 83:531-537, 1952.

Grayson, C. E., and Black, H. A.: Myelography, diagnostic value in lesions of lumbar intervertebral discs with variations in technique, Calif. Med. 70:464-471, 1949.

Greenberg, A. D., and Flanigan, S.: A follow-up evaluation of lumbar disc surgery, Conn. Med. 31:848-849, 1967.

Greenwood, J., Jr.: Protruded intervertebral disc, Med. Rec. Ann. 40:1289-1290, 1946.

Greenwood, J., Jr.: Protruded intervertebral

disc; diagnosis, treatment, and results, Arizona Med. **4**:33-36, 1947.

Greenwood, J., Jr., McGuire, T. H., and Kimbell, F.: Study of causes of failure in herniated intervertebral disc operation; analysis of 67 reoperated cases, J. Neurosurg. **9**:15-20, 1952.

Greitz, T., Liliequist, B., and Muller, R.: Cervical vertebral phlebography, Acta Radiol. **57**:353-365, 1962.

Gresham, J. L., and Miller, R.: Evaluation of the lumbar spine by diskography and its use in selection of proper treatment of the herniated disk syndrome, Clin. Orthop. **67**:29-41, 1969.

Grewal, K. S., and Mohan, P.: Syndrome of protruded intervertebral disc in lumbar region, Indian J. Med. Sci. **5**:716-718, 1951.

Griffiths, D. L.: Sciatica and intervertebral disk, Clin. J. **76**:127-133, 1947.

Gurdjian, E. S., and Webster, J. E.: Lumbar herniations of nucleus pulposus; analysis of 196 operated cases, Amer. J. Surg. **76**:235-243, 1948.

Gurdjian, E. S., Ostrowski, A. Z., Hardy, W. G., Lindner, D. W., and Thomas, L. M.: Results of operative treatment of protruded and ruptured lumbar discs based on 1176 operative cases with 82 percent follow-up of 3 to 13 years, J. Neurosurg. **18**:783-791, 1961.

Gurdjian, E. S., Webster, J. E., Ostrowski, A. Z., Hardy, W. G., Lindner, D. W., and Thomas, L. M.: Herniated lumbar intervertebral discs—analysis of 1176 operated cases, J. Trauma **1**:158-176, 1961.

Gustilo, R. H., and Walker, A. E.: Herniated lumbar nucleus pulposus; diagnosis and surgical management, Philipp. J. Surg. **5**:99-110, 1950.

Haas, S. L.: Fusion of vertebrae following resection of intervertebral disc, J. Bone Joint Surg. **28**:544-549, 1946.

Haas, S. L.: Resection of intervertebral disk through posterior approach, Arch. Surg. **59**:1261-1264, 1949.

Hadley, J.: Exercises in the treatment of lumbar intervertebral disc protrusions, Physiotherapy **50**:296-299, 1964.

Hadley, L. A.: Constriction of intervertebral foramen; cause of nerve root pressure, J.A.M.A. **140**:473-476, 1949.

Hadley, L. A.: Intervertebral foramen studies; foramen encroachment associated with disc herniation, J. Neurosurg. **7**:347-351, 1950.

Hadley, L. A.: Intervertebral joint subluxation, bony impingement and foramen encroachment with nerve root changes, Amer. J. Roentgen. **65**:377-402, 1951.

Hafner, R. H. V.: Case illustrating hazards of manipulative treatment in lumbosacral disk protrusions, Brit. Med. J. **1**:361-362, 1952.

Hafner, R. H., James, C. D., and Robertshaw, R.: Induced muscle relaxation in the treatment of lumbar intervertebral disc lesions, Postgrad. Med. **42**:36-40, 1966.

Haggart, G. E., and Terheyden, W. A., Jr.: Present management of disk lesions in lumbar spine, Surg. Clin. N. Amer. **35**:859-864, 1955.

Haimovich, H.: Clinical observations and evaluation of conservative treatment of acute low back pain due to disc lesions, Acta Orthop. Scand. **29**:98-107, 1959.

Halbstein, B. M.: Operative treatment of low back pain, J. Med. Soc. New Jersey **49**:496-500, 1952.

Haley, J. C., and Perry, J. H.: Protrusions of intervertebral discs; study of their distribution, characteristics and effects on nervous system, Amer. J. Surg. **80**:394-404, 1950.

Hall, H.: Review of 93 laminectomies for low backache and crural pain, J. Roy. Army Med. Corps **91**:156-157, 1948.

Hallock, H.: Fusion versus interlaminer excision alone in lumbar disk lesions, New York J. Med. **52**:3001-3002, 1952.

Hamby, W. B., and Glasser, H. T.: Replacement of spinal intervertebral disc with locally polymerizing methyl methacrylate: experimental study of effects upon tissues and report of a small clinical series, J. Neurosurg. **16**:311-313, 1959.

Hanraets, P. R. M. J.: The degenerative back and its differential diagnosis, Amsterdam, 1959, Elsevier Publishing Co.

Hansen, H. J.: Pathologic-anatomical interpretation of disc degeneration in dogs, Acta Orthop. Scand. **20**:280-293, 1951.

Hansen, H. J., and Ullberg, S.: Uptake of S35 in the intervertebral discs after injection of S35-sulfate; an autoradiographic study, Acta Orthop. Scand. **30**:84-90, 1960.

Hansen, J. W.: Postoperative management in lumbar disc protrusions. I. Indications, method and results. II. Follow-up on a trained and an untrained group of patients, Acta Orthop. Scand. supp. **71**:1-47, 1964.

Hansen, J. W.: Statometric studies on patients operated upon for slipped disc in the lumbar region, Acta Orthop. Scand. **34**:225-238, 1964.

Happey, F., Wiseman, A., and Naylor, A.: Polysaccharide content of the prolapsed nucleus pulposus of the human intervertebral disk, Nature **192**:580, 1962.

Harbison, S. P.: Major vascular complications of intervertebral disc surgery, Ann. Surg. **140**:342-348, 1954.

Hardin, C. A., and Allen, M.: Arteriovenous fistula; report of case developing after operation for ruptured intervertebral disc and successfully repaired homograft, J. Kansas Med. Soc. **59**:93-95, 1958.

Hardy, W. G., Lindner, D. W., Thomas, L. M., and Gurdjian, E. S.: Conditions affecting the cervical brachial neural and vascular components to be differentiated from cervical disk and joint disease, Clin. Orthop. **27**:78-82, 1963.

Hargrave-Wilson, W.: Conservative treatment of low backache, E. Afr. Med. J. **30**:377-383, 1953.

Harmon, P. H.: Results from treatment of sciatica due to lumbar disc protrusion, Amer. J. Surg. **80**:829-840, 1950.

Harmon, P. H.: Saline injection test applied to lower lumbar disc degeneration: comparison to Pantopaque myelography, Ann. Surg. **156**:767-775, 1962.

Harmon, P. H.: Anterior excision and vertebral body fusion operation for intervertebral disk syndromes of the lower lumbar spine: three-to-five year results in 244 cases, Clin. Orthop. **26**:107-127, 1963.

Harris, R. I., and Macnab, I.: Structural changes in lumbar intervertebral discs; relationship to low back pain and sciatica, J. Bone Joint Surg. **36-B**:304-322, 1954.

Hart, G. M.: Circumscribed serous spinal arachnoiditis simulating protruded lumbar intervertebral disc, Ann. Surg. **148**:266-270, 1958.

Hasner, E., et al.: Degeneration of lumbar intervertebral discs, Amer. J. Phys. Med. **31**:441-449, 1952.

Haynes, W. G., and Ross, G. L.: Near electrocution as cause of protrusion of intervertebral disc; case report, Southern Med. J. **40**:874-875, 1947.

Hazouri, L. A.: Ruptured intervertebral disc syndrome, J. Med. Ass. Georgia **43**:30-32, 1954.

Hegarty, W. M., and Elkins, C. W.: Management of herniated intervertebral lumbar disc, Ohio Med. J. **49**:33-37, 1953.

Hellstadius, A.: Some cases of paradiscal defects in anterior portion of vertebral body with remarks on pathogenesis of lesions in question, Acta Orthop. Scand. **17**:50-69, 1947.

Hellstadius, A.: Experiences gained from spondylosyndesis operations with H-shaped bone transplantations in case of degeneration of discs in lumbar back, Acta Orthop. Scand. **24**:207-215, 1955.

Henderson, R. S.: Treatment of lumbar intervertebral disk protrusion; assessment of conservative measures, Brit. Med. J. **2**:597-598, 1952.

Hendry, N. G.: The hydration of the nucleus pulposus and its relation to intervertebral disc derangement, J. Bone Joint Surg. **40-B**:132-144, 1958.

Hepburn, H. H.: Protruded intervertebral disc, Canad. Med. Ass. J. **57**:273-276, 1947.

Hepburn, H. H.: Herniated intervertebral disc with sciatic syndrome, Canad. Med. Ass. J. **69**:55-60, 1953.

Herzberger, E. E., Kindschi, L. G., Bear, N. E., and Chandler, A.: Treatment of cervical disc disease and cervical spine injury by anterior interbody fusion. A report on early results in 72 cases, Zbl. Neurochir. **23**:215-227, 1963.

Herzog, J. B.: Surgical results in lumbar disc protrusions, J. Amer. Osteopath. Ass. **62**:27-29, 1962.

Hirsch, C.: Intervertebral foraminotomy, Acta Chir. Scand. **94**:75-80, 1946.

Hirsch, C.: Instability in degeneration of lumbar disk; anatomic study, Nord. Med. **38**:1252-1254, 1948.

Hirsch, C.: The reaction of intervertebral discs to compression forces, J. Bone Joint Surg. **37-A**:1188-1196, 1955.

Hirsch, C.: Exposure of ruptured lumbar discs; a technical discussion, Acta Orthop. Scand. **28**:76-80, 1958.

Hirsch, C.: Cervical disk rupture; diagnosis and therapy, Acta Orthop. Scand. **30**:172-186, 1960.

Hirsch, C., and Nachemson, A.: New observations on mechanical behavior of lumbar discs, Acta Orthop. Scand. **23**:254-283, 1954.

Hirsch, C., and Nachemson, A.: The reliability of lumbar disk surgery, Clin. Orthop. **29**:189-195, 1963.

Hirsch, C., and Schajowicz, F.: Studies on structural changes in lumbar annulus fibrosus, Acta Orthop. Scand. **22**:184-231, 1953.

Hirsch, E., Paulson, S., Sylven, B., and Shellman, O.: Biophysical and physiological investigations on cartilage and other mesenchymal tissues; characteristics of human nuclei pulposi during aging, Acta Orthop. Scand. **22**:175-183, 1953.

Hoeberechts, P. M. J. J. P.: Surgical technique in herniated intervertebral disc. Canad. Med. Ass. J. **72**:926-927, 1955.

Hoen, T. I., Anderson, R. K., and Clare, F. B.: Symposium on neurosurgery; lesions of intervertebral disks, Surg. Clin. N. Amer. **28**:456-466, 1948.

Hoen, T. I., and Clare, F. B.: Operative positions in neurosurgery, U. S. Naval Med. Bull. **49**:129-136, 1949.

Hoen, T. I., Druckemiller, W. H., and Cook, A. W.: Injection of lumbar intervertebral disks, diagnostic method, U. S. Armed Forces Med. J. **2**:1067-1074, 1951.

Höerlein, B. F.: Intervertebral disc protrusions in the dog, Amer. J. Vet. Res. **14**:260-283, 1953.

Höerlein, B. F.: Further evaluation of the treatment of disc protrusion paraplegia in the dog, J. Amer. Vet. Med. Ass. **129**:495-502, 1956.

Holm, K. L.: Herniated nucleus pulposus, Med. Bull., Chief Surgeon, European Command (No. 6) **2**:27-32, 1947.

Holmes, J. M., and Sworn, B. R.: Sciatic "neuritis," Brit. Med. J. **2**:350-351, 1945.

Holmes, J. M., and Sworn, B. R.: Lumbosacral root pain, Brit. Med. J. **1**:946-948, 1946.

Holscher, E. C.: Vascular complication of disc surgery, J. Bone Joint Surg. **30-A**:968-970, 1948.

Holstein, A., and Lewis, G. B.: Laminectomy and fusion for disc lesions, Calif. Med. **86**:91-92, 1957.

Hood, L. B., and Chrisman, D.: Intermittent pelvic traction in the treatment of the ruptured intervertebral disk, Phys. Ther. **48**:21-30, 1968.

Hooff, A. van den: Histological age changes in the anulus fibrosus of the human intervertebral disk; with a discussion of the problems of disk herniation, Gerontologia **9**:136-149, 1964.

Hook, O., Lindvall, H., and Astrom, K. E.: Cervical disk protrusions with compression of the spinal cord; report of a case, Neurology **10**:834-841, 1960.

Hopkyns, J. C. W.: An unusual trophic ulcer, Brit. Med. J. **2**:905, 1948.

Horton, R. E.: Arteriovenous fistula following operation for prolapsed intervertebral disk, Brit. J. Surg. **49**:77-80, 1961.

Horwitz, T.: Some pathologic considerations in the diagnosis of lumbar intervertebral disk lesions, Bull. Hosp. Joint Dis. **25**:21-29, 1964.

Hoytema, G. T., and Oostrom, J.: The operation for herniation of the nucleus pulposus with intervertebral body fusion, Arch. Chir. Neerl. **13**:71-80, 1961.

Hudgins, W. R.: The predictive value of myelography in the diagnosis of ruptured lumbar discs, J. Neurosurg. **32**:152-162, 1970.

Hufnagel, C. A., Walsh, B. J., and Conrad, P. W.: Iliac-caval arteriovenous fistula following operation for herniated disc, Angiology **12**:579-582, 1961.

Hughes, R. R.: Retropulsed intervertebral disk producing Froin's syndrome; report of case, Lancet **2**:401, 1945.

Hulme, A.: The surgical approach to thoracic intervertebral disc protrusions, J. Neurol. Neurosurg. Psychiat. **23**:133-137, 1960.

Hult, L.: Retroperitoneal disc fenestration in low-back pain and sciatica; preliminary report, Acta Orthop. Scand. **20**:342-348, 1951.

Hulten, O.: Intradural gelegener Diskusprolaps, Acta Chir. Scand. **92**:228-230, 1945.

Hunt, W. E., and Paul, S.: Herniated cervical and lumbar discs, Nebraska Med. J. **5**:778-783, 1969.

Hunt, W. E., and Paul, S.: Herniated cervical and lumbar discs; a discussion of clinical findings and diagnostic procedures, Ohio Med. J. **65**:583-587, 1969.

Hunter, A. R.: Anesthesia for operations in vertebral canal, Anesthesiology **11**:367-373, 1950.

Hyndman, O. R.: Pathologic intervertebral disc and its consequences; contribution to cause and treatment of chronic pain low in back and to subject of herniating intervertebral disc, Arch. Surg. **53**:247-297, 1946.

Ingebrigtsen, R.: Indications for spinal fusion immediately following removal of protruded nucleus pulposus, Acta Orthop. Scand. **22**:25-35, 1952.

Inman, V. T., and Saunders, J. B. de C. M.: Anatomico-physiological aspects of injuries to intervertebral disc, J. Bone Joint Surg. **29**:461-475, 1947.

Irsigler, F. J.: The place of neurosurgery in lumbar intervertebral disc herniations, Neurochirurgia **7**:157-165, 1964.

Jack, E. A.: Sciatica and intervertebral disc, Rheumatism **3**:122-125, 1947.

Jackson, H.: Surgical aspects of spinal condition, Postgrad. Med. **23**:244-248, 1947.

Jackson, H.: Association between certain anatomical facts, normal and morbid, and symptomatology of intervertebral disc protrusions in lumbar region; Hunterian lecture, Ann. Roy. Coll. Surg. Eng. **2**:273-284, 1948.

Jadeson, W. J.: Rehabilitation of dogs with intervertebral disk lesions, J. Amer. Vet. Med. Ass. **138**:411-423, 1961.

Jaeger, R.: Injury to intervertebral disk with sciatic neuralgia and backache, Penn. Med. J. **50**:1164-1169, 1947.

Jaeger, R.: Injury of the lumbar intervertebral disk: treatment by intercorporeal fusion through complete removal, Penn. Med. **62**:966-968, 1959.

James, A., and Nisbet, N. W.: Posterior intervertebral fusion of lumbar spine; preliminary report of new operation, J. Bone Joint Surg. **35-B**:181-187, 1953.

James, U.: Collapsed intervertebral discs following lumbar puncture, Proc. Roy. Soc. Med. **39**:134-135, 1946.

Jaslow, I. A.: Intercorporal bone graft in spinal fusion after disc removal, Surg. Gynec. Obstet. **82**:215-218, 1946.

Jelsma, F.: Protruded intervertebral disc, Kentucky Med. J. **45**:401-405, 1947.

Jenkner, F. L., Foltz, E. L., and Ward, A. A., Jr.: Experimental intervertebral fusion using basic calcium phosphate, J. Neurosurg. **10**:443-452, 1953.

Jennett, W. B.: A study of 25 cases of compression of the cauda equina by prolapsed intervertebral discs, J. Neurol. Neurosurg. Psychiat. **19**:109-116, 1956.

Jirout, J., and Kunc, Z.: Traumatic herniation of the thoracic intervertebral disc, Acta Neurochir. **8**:88-93, 1960.

Jocson, C. T.: Excision of lumbar intervertebral discs through the lateral approach, J. Philipp. Med. Ass. **38**:838-842, 1962.

Joffe, B.: Circulatory complication from disc surgery, GP **25**:100-101, 1962.

Johnson, R. W., Jr., Hillman, J. W., and Southwick, W. O.: Importance of direct surgical attack upon lesions of vertebral bodies, particularly in Pott's disease, J. Bone Joint Surg. **35-A**:17-25, 1953.

Jonck, L. M.: The mechanical disturbances resulting from lumbar disc space narrowing, J. Bone Joint Surg. **43-B**:362-375, 1961.

Jones, H. T.: Low back pain from orthopedic standpoint, Calif. Med. **68**:57-64, 1948.

Jones, K. G.: Lumbar intervertebral disc disease in the elderly, J. Arkansas Med. Soc. **65**:465-473, 1969.

Jones, K. G., and Barnett, H. C.: Use of hydrocortisone in spinal surgery, Southern Med. J. **48**:617-623, 1955.

Jones, O. W., Jr.: Lumbar intervertebral disc problem, Industr. Med. Surg. **23**:112-115, 1954.

Josey, A. I., and Murphey, F.: Ruptured intervertebral disk simulating angina pectoris, J.A.M.A. **131**:581-587, 1946.

Judovich, B. D.: Lumbar traction therapy and dissipated force factors, J. Lancet **74**:411-414, 1954.

Judovich, B. D.: Lumbar traction therapy—elimination of physical factors that prevent lumbar stretch, J.A.M.A. **159**:549-550, 1955.

Kabat, H., and Saltzman, A.: Electromyography; aid to diagnosis of amyotrophic lateral sclerosis and motor root compression syndromes; with case reports, Rhode Island Med. J. **41**:617-620, 1958.

Kalima, T.: Simple, thorough operative technic for excochleation of disc herniation, J. Int. Coll. Surg. **9**:531-535, 1946.

Kallio, K. E.: Rupture of the lumbar interspinous ligament, diagnosed by contrast-medium x-ray and reconstructed by free cutis graft, Bull. Hosp. Joint Dis. **21**:198-199, 1960.

Kambin, P., Smith, J. M., and Hoerner, E. F.: Myelography and myography in diagnosis of herniated intervertebral disk; use in confirming clinical findings, J.A.M.A. **181**:472-475, 1962.

Kane, C. A., and Lane, G. M.: Symposium on specific methods of treatment: diagnosis and management of herniated disks, Med. Clin. N. Amer. **39**:1463-1482, 1955.

Kang, S. R.: Myography of the multifidus muscle, Acta Radiol. **57**:273-279, 1962.

Kaplan, A.: Neurosurgical aspects of low back pain, Bull. Hosp. Joint Dis. **7**:99-108, 1946.

Kaplan, A.: Peroneal palsy due to giant herniated intervertebral disc, Bull. Hosp. Joint Dis. **9**:124-130, 1948.

Kaplan, A.: Herniated intervertebral discs producing contralateral symptoms and signs; report of 2 cases, Bull. Hosp. Joint Dis. **10**:207-216, 1949.

Kaplan, A., and Umansky, A. L.: Myelographic defects of intervertebral herniated discs simulating cauda equina neoplasms, Amer. J. Surg. **81**:262-278, 1951.

Karr, H. H.: The problem of the ruptured intervertebral disk, Southern Med. J. **53**:341-345, 1960.

Keats, S.: Management of pain associated with disturbances of intervertebral disc, J. Med. Soc. New Jersey **46**:376-379, 1949.

Keck, C.: Discography; technique and interpretation, Arch. Surg. **80**:580-585, 1960.

Keegan, J. J.: Variation of symptoms with herniation of intervertebral discs, Nebraska Med. J. **43**:191-194, 1958.

Keegan, J. J.: Relations of nerve roots to abnormalities of lumbar and cervical portions of spine, Arch. Surg. **55**:246-270, 1947.

Keegan, J. J.: Alterations of lumbar curve related to posture and seating, J. Bone Joint Surg. **35-A**:589-603, 1953.

Keet, P. W. J.: Sciatic and analogous root pains and their treatment by paravertebral injection, S. Afr. J. Med. Sci. **28**:65-68, 1954.

Kelley, J. H., Voris, D. C., Svien, H. J., and Ghormley, R. K.: Multiple operations for protruded intervertebral disk, Proc. Staff Meet. Mayo Clin. **29**:546-550, 1954; correction **29**:581, 1954.

Kelly, M.: Is pain due to pressure on nerves? Spinal tumors and the intervertebral disk, Neurology **6**:32-36, 1956.

Kendall, D.: Aetiology, diagnosis and treatment of prolapsed intervertebral disk with review of 300 cases of sciatica, Quart. J. Med. **16**:157-179, 1947.

Kennedy, F., Hyde, B., and Kaufman, S.: Herniated disc simulating cord tumor, J. Nerv. Ment. Dis. **108**:32-35, 1948.

Kern, C. E.: Delayed death following disk surgery, Texas Med. **50**:158-160, 1954.

Kessler, L. A., and Stern, W. Z.: Posterior migration of a herniated disc, Radiology **76**:104-106, 1961.

Kettunen, K., and Salenius, P.: Peridurography in the lumbosacral region for the diagnosis of protruded intervertebral discs,

Ann. Chir. Gynaec. Fenn. **52:**709-719, 1963.

Key, J. A.: Conservative and operative treatment of lesions of intervertebral discs in low back, Surgery **17:**291-303, 1945.

Key, J. A.: Intervertebral disc lesions are most common causes of low back pain with or without sciatica, Ann. Surg. **121:**534-544, 1945; Trans. Southern Surg. Ass. **56:**150-169, 1945.

Key, J. A.: Diagnosis and treatment of intervertebral disc lesions in low back, J. Okla. Med. Ass. **43:**198-204, 1950.

Key, J. A.: Intervertebral-disc lesions in children and adolescents, J. Bone Joint Surg. **32-A:**97-102, 1950.

Key, J. A.: Indications for operation in disc lesions in lumbosacral spine, Ann. Surg. **135:**886-891, 1952.

Key, J. A.: Intervertebral disk: anatomy, physiology, and pathology, Amer. Acad. Orthop. Surg. Lect. **11:**101-107, 1954.

Key, J. A., and Ford, L. T.: Experimental intervertebral disc lesions, J. Bone Joint Surg. **30-A:**621-630, 1948.

Key, J. A., and Ford, L. T.: Management of patient with ruptured intervertebral disc in low back, Chicago Med. Soc. Bull. **55:**434-438, 1952.

King, A. B.: Back pain due to loose facets of lower lumbar vertebrae, Bull. Johns Hopkins Hosp. **97:**271-283, 1955.

King, A. B.: Phantom sciatica, Arch. Neurol. Psychiat. **76:**72-74, 1956.

King, M. K.: Rupture of lower lumbar intervertebral disks, Amer. J. Surg. **72:**161-165, 1946.

Kirstein, L.: After-examination of operated and non-operated cases with "clinical symptoms of herniated disc," Acta Med. Scand. **120:**93-106, 1945.

Knape, H.: Bezitramide, an orally active analgesic. An investigation on pain following operations for lumbar disc protrusion (preliminary report), Brit. J. Anaesth. **42:**325-328, 1970.

Knighton, R. S., and Hitselberger, W. E.: A study of patients ten to seventeen years following operation for herniated nucleus pulposus, Western J. Surg. **72:**134-138, 1964.

Knutsson, B.: Electromyographic studies in the diagnosis of lumbar disc herniations, Acta Orthop. Scand. **28:**290-299, 1959.

Knutsson, B.: How often do the neurological signs disappear after the operation for a herniated disc? Acta Orthop. Scand. **32:**352-356, 1962.

Knutsson, B., and Wiberg, G.: On surgically treated herniated intervertebral discs, Acta Orthop. Scand. **28:**108-123, 1958.

Knutsson, F.: Slight and severe instability states of lumbar spine in disc degeneration, Nord. Med. **31:**1875-1876, 1946.

Knutsson, F.: Myelogram following operation for herniated disc, Acta Radiol. **32:**60-65, 1949.

Knutsson, F.: Lumbar myelography with water-soluble contrast in cases of disc prolapse, Acta Orthop. Scand. **20:**294-302, 1951.

Koch, D. M.: A personal experience with pain, Amer. J. Surg. **59:**1434-1435, 1959.

Kondo, E., et al.: Osteoplastic laminectomy for lumbar disc protrusion, Arch. Jap. Chir. **23:**287-294, 1954.

Kondo, S., Ando, T., Ikeura, T., et al.: A statistical study on the diagnosis of lumbar intervertebral disc herniation, Bull. Osaka Med. Sch. **15:**38-45, 1969.

Kontturi, M.: Investigations into bladder dysfunction in prolapse of lumbar intervertebral disc, Ann. Chir. Gynaec. Fenn. 57 (supp.):1-53, 1968.

Kontturi, M., Harviainen, S., and Larmi, T. K.: Atonic bladder in lumbar disk herniation, Acta Chir. Scand. supp. 357:232+, 1966.

Koskinen, E. V.: The value of the disc operation in prolonged disabling sciatica; a clinical study with an evaluation of results and symptoms based on the follow-up examination of 104 cases, Ann. Chir. Gynaec. Fenn, **46:**1-66, 1957.

Kovacs, A.: Herniated disks and vertebral ligaments on native roentgenograms, Acta Radiol. **32:**287-303, 1949.

Kremer, M., and Furlong, R.: Lesions of intervertebral discs, Trans. Med. Soc. London (1953-1954) **70:**211-221, 1954.

Kristoff, F. V., and Odom, G. L.: Ruptured disc in cervical region (causing root and cord compression); 20 cases, Arch. Surg. **54:**287-304, 1947.

Kristoff, F. V., and Odom, G. L.: Variations in syndrome of ruptured intervertebral disc in lumbar region, Surgery **22:**83-93, 1947.

Kugelberg, E., and Peterson, I.: Muscle weakness and wasting in sciatica due to fourth lumbar or lumbosacral disc herniations, J. Neurosurg. **7:**270-277, 1950.

Kuhn, H. H., and Neill, R. G.: Results of removal of ruptured intervertebral discs and combined disc-fusion operations; analysis of 288 operations, Southern Med. J. **39:**745-750, 1946.

Kumpuris, M.: Postoperative herniated nucleus pulposus, Phys. Ther. Rev. **39:**804-806, 1959.

LaFia, D. J.: Ruptured lumbar intervertebral disk symdrome caused by metastatic disease, Rhode Island Med. J. **38:**212-213, 1955.

Laitinen, L.: Defects of the lumbar interspinous ligaments, Ann. Chir. Gynaec. Fenn. **51:**486-491, 1962.

Lambert, C. N.: Relation of occupational strains to "disc syndrome," J. Int. Coll. Surg. **17**:860-863, 1952.

Lane, J. D., Jr., and Moore, E. S., Jr.: Transperitoneal approach to intervertebral disc in lumbar area, Ann. Surg. **127**:537-551, 1948.

Lang, E. F., Jr.: Cervical spondylosis, Postgrad. Med. **33**:58-64, 1963.

Lange, J.: Abrodil myelography in protrusion of intervertebral disk, Acta Chir. Scand. **104**:181-187, 1952.

Lange, J., and Edgaard, H.: Abrodil myelography in herniated disk in lumbar region, Radiology **57**:186-192, 1951.

Lanigan, J. P.: Neurosurgical relief of pain, Irish J. Med. Sci., pp. 517-522, 1947.

Lannin, D. R.: Intervertebral disc lesions in teenage group, Minn. Med. **37**:136-137, 1954.

Lansche, W. E., and Ford, L. T.: Correlation of the myelogram with clinical and operative findings in lumbar disc lesions, J. Bone Joint Surg. **42-A**:193-206, 1960.

Larsen, E. H., and Kristoffersen, K.: Follow-up of patients submitted to operation for herniation of lumbar intervertebral disc, Acta Psychiat. Neurol. Scand. supp. 108:217-224, 1956.

Larson, C. B.: Medical progress; orthopedic surgery; problem of intervertebral disc, New Eng. J. Med. **232**:137-139, 1945.

Larson, C. B.: Low back pain, Postgrad. Med. **26**:142-149, 1959.

LaSorte, A. F., and Brown, N.: Ruptured anterior nucleus pulposus between T1 and T2 causing a discrete esophageal defect and minimal dysphagia, Amer. J. Surg. **98**:631-634, 1959.

Leader, S. A., and Rassell, M. J.: Value of Pantopaque (ethyl iodophenylundecylate, iodized oil) myelography in diagnosis of herniation of nucleus pulposus in lumbosacral spine; report of 500 cases, Amer. J. Roentgen. **69**:231-241, 1953.

Leao, L.: Intradiscal injection of hydrocortisone and prednisolone in the treatment of low back pain, Rheumatism **16**:72-77, 1960.

Leavens, M. E., and Bradford, F. K.: Ruptured intervertebral disc; report of case with defect in anterior annulus fibrosus, J. Neurosurg. **10**:544-546, 1953.

Lee, D. G.: The arterial supply of the intervertebral disk of the domestic cat (Felix domestica) from fetal life to old age, Amer. J. Vet. Res. **23**:1072-1077, 1962.

Lehmann, J. F., and Brunner, G. D.: A device for the application of heavy lumbar traction: its mechanical effects, Arch. Phys. Med. **39**:696-700, 1958.

Lehmann, P. O.: Protruded intervertebral disc (report on 60 operative cases), Bull. Vancouver Med. Ass. **22**:56-60; Canad. Med. Serv. **3**:244-250, 1946.

Lehmann, P. O.: Protruded intervertebral discs, Treat. Serv. Bull. **3**:3-9, 1948.

Leigh, A. D.: Prolapsed intervertebral disc, Postgrad. Med. **23**:141-150, 1947.

Lenhard, R. E.: End-result study of intervertebral disc, J. Bone Joint Surg. **29**:425-428, 1947.

Lenshoek, C. H.: Infection of intervertebral disk following operation for protrusion of nucleus pulposus, Arch. Chir. Neerl. **8**:57-66, 1956.

LeVay, D.: A survey of surgical management of lumbar disc prolapse in the United Kingdom and Erie, Lancet **1**:1211-1213, 1967.

Levy, L. F.: Lumbar intervertebral disc disease in Africans, J. Neurosurg. **26**:31-34, 1967.

Levy, R. W., Payzant, A. R., and Karr, H. H.: Pantopaque myelography in ruptured intervertebral disk: correlation with operative findings, New Orleans Med. Surg. J. **103**:390-393, 1951.

Lewey, F. H.: Mechanism of intervertebral disc protrusion, Surg. Gynec. Obstet. **88**:592-602, 1949.

Lewin, P.: Intervertebral disk syndrome, J. Int. Coll. Surg. **11**:137-147, 1948.

Lewin, W.: Sciatica and prolapsed intervertebral disc, Med. Press **214**:392-395, 1945.

Ley, E. B., and Thurston, W. D.: Retroperitoneal approach to lumbar disc, Rocky Mountain Med. J. **51**:121-123, 1954.

Lie, T. A., and Smet, H. L. de: Major vascular injuries following operations for protruded lumbar discs, Psychiat. Neurol. Neurochir. **71**:71-75, 1968.

Lin, T. H., and Cooper, I. S.: Association of parkinsonism and other neurologic disorders, New York J. Med. **63**:2088-2094, 1963.

Lindblom, A.: The roentgenographic appearance of injuries to the intervertebral discs, Acta Radiol. **45**:129-132, 1956.

Lindblom, K.: Roentgen diagnosis of disk prolapse, Nord. Med. **30**:1173-1176, 1946.

Lindblom, K.: Diagnostic puncture of intervertebral disks in sciatica, Acta Orthop. Scand. **17**:231-239, 1948.

Lindblom, K.: Technique and results in myelography and disc puncture, Acta Radiol. **34**:321-330, 1950.

Lindblom, K.: Backache and its relation to ruptures of intervertebral disks, Radiology **57**:710-718, 1951.

Lindblom, K.: Discography of dissecting transosseous ruptures of intervertebral discs in lumbar region, Acta Radiol. **36**:12-16, 1951.

Lindblom, K.: Technique and results of diagnostic disc puncture and injection (discography) in lumbar region, Acta Orthop. Scand. **20:**315-326, 1951.

Lindblom, K.: Intervertebral-disc degeneration considered as a pressure atrophy, J. Bone Joint Surg. **39-A:**933-945, 1957.

Lindblom, K., and Hultquist, G. T.: Absorption of protruded disc tissue, J. Bone Joint Surg. **32-A:**557-560, 1950.

Lindgren, S.: Some problems concerning herniated intervertebral disk from clinical point of view, Acta Chir. Scand. **98:**295-314, 1949.

Lindon, L.: Some problems of backache and sciatica, Med. J. Aust. **2:**345-347, 1946.

Linton, R. R., and White, P. D.: Arteriovenous fistula between right common iliac artery and inferior vena cava; case of its occurrence following operation for ruptured intervertebral disk with cure by operation, Arch. Surg. **50:**6-13, 1945.

Lipkin, E.: Protrusion of intervertebral disk, Mich. Med. **51:**1216-1218, 1952.

Lodin, H.: Myelography with Pantopaque in the diagnosis of cervical disk herniation, Acta Orthop. Scand. **30:**187-201, 1960.

Logan, E.: Counter-torque suspension; a conservative means of treatment for lumbar disc herniation, Physiotherapy **44:**71-74, 1958.

Logan, T.: The treatment of intervertebral disc protrusions with salt, J. Coll. Gen. Pract. **4:**96-100, 1961.

Logue, V.: Treatment of lumbar intervertebral disc prolapse, Postgrad. Med. **29:**234-242, 1953.

Loopesko, E.: Conservative treatment of industrial intervertebral disc injuries, Industr. Med. Surg. **18:**457-461, 1949.

Loughlen, I., and Anderson, R.: The ligamentum flavum—why destroy it? Amer. J. Orthop. **5:**94-95, 1963.

Louison, R., and Barber, J. B.: Massive herniation of lumbar discs with compression of the cauda equina—a surgical emergency; report of 2 cases, J. Nat. Med. Ass. **60:**188-190, 1968.

Love, J. G.: Protruded intervertebral disk, Surg. Clin. N. Amer. **26:**997-1006, 1946.

Love, J. G.: Disc factor in low-back pain with or without sciatica, J. Bone Joint Surg. **29:**438-447, 1947.

Love, J. G.: Protruded intervertebral disks as cause of disabling pain and paralysis, Virginia Med. Monthly **74:**398-400, 1947.

Love, J. G., and Emmett, J. L.: "Asymptomatic" protruded lumbar disk as a cause of urinary retention: preliminary report, Mayo Clin. Proc. **42:**249-257, 1967.

Love, J. G., and Rivers, M. H.: Protruded cervical disk simulating spinal-cord tumor: report of a case, Mayo Clin. Proc. **36:**344-346, 1961.

Love, J. G., and Rivers, M. H.: Intractable pain due to associated protruded inter-

vertebral disk and intraspinal neoplasm; report of cases, Neurology **12:**60-64, 1962.

Love, J. G., and Rivers, M. H.: Spinal cord tumors simulating protruded intervertebral disks, J.A.M.A. **179:**878-881, 1962.

Lowry, J. G.: An operative series of lumbar intervertebral discs, Ulster Med. J. **32:**208-209, 1963.

Luck, J. V.: Discogenic syndromes—factors in differential diagnosis, Instruct. Lect. Amer. Acad. Orthop. Surg. **18:**35-40, 1961.

Lund, P. C.: Hypobaric Pontocaine (tetracaine) spinal anesthesia for exploration for extruded nucleus pulposus, Anesth. Analg. **27:**301-313, 1948.

Luyendijk, W.: Canalography. Roentgenological examination of the peridural space in the lumbosacral part of the vertebral canal, J. Belg. Radiol. **46:**236-254, 1963.

Lyerly, J. G.: Dislocated intervertebral disc of lumbar region, J. Florida Med. Ass. **33:**377-382, 1947.

Lyerly, J. G., and Grizzard, V. T.: Dislocated disc of lumbar region; statistical analysis of series of cases, Southern Surg. **14:**755-765, 1948.

Lyons, A. E., and Wise, B. L.: Subarachnoid rupture of intervertebral disc fragments, J. Neurosurg. **18:**242-244, 1961.

Lyons, H., Jones, E., and Quinn, F. E., et al.: Protein-polysaccharide complexes of normal and herniated human intervertebral discs, Proc. Soc. Exp. Biol. Med. **115:**610-615, 1964.

MacCarty, W. C., Jr., and Lane, F. W., Jr.: Pitfalls of myelography, Radiology **65:**663-670, 1955.

MacDonald, A.: Low back strains, manipulations and "slipped discs," New Zeal. Med. J. **58:**359-361, 1959.

Macey, H. B.: Derangement of disk; possible pain mechanisms, Texas Med. **47:**695-699, 1951.

MacGee, E. E.: Protruded lumbar disc in a 9-year-old boy, J. Pediat. **73:**418-419, 1968.

Mack, E. W.: Electromyographic observations on postoperative disc patient, J. Neurosurg. **8:**469-472, 1951.

Mack, J. R.: Major vascular injuries incident to intervertebral disk surgery, Amer. Surg. **22:**752-763, 1956.

Magill, C. D.: The aggravated EMG—a new sign in lumbar disk lesions, Rocky Mountain Med. J. **66:**32-34, 1969.

Magnuson, P. B.: Intervertebral discs, Amer. J. Surg. **67:**228-236, 1945.

Malinsky, J.: The ontogenetic development of nerve terminations in the intervertebral discs of man (histology of intervertebral discs, 11th communication), Acta Anat. **38:**96-113, 1959.

Malis, L. I., Newman, C. M., and Wolf, B. S.: Full-column technic in lumbar disk myelography, Radiology 60:18-27, 1953.

Malloch, J. D.: Acute retention due to intervertebral disc prolapse, Brit. J. Urol. 37:578, 1965.

Malmros, R.: Clinical syndromes in protrusion of lumbar intervertebral discs, Acta Psychiat. Neurol. Scand. supp. 108:255-264, 1956.

Mandell, A. J.: Lumbosacral intervertebral disc disease in children, Calif. Med. 93:307-308, 1960.

Marble, H. C., and Bishop, W. A.: Intervertebal disc injury; analysis from industrial standpoint, J. Industr. Hyg. Toxicol. 27:103-109, 1945.

Marble, H. C., and Bishop, W. A.: Intervertebal disc injury; analysis of 113 industrial cases, J. Industr. Hyg. Toxicol. 31:46-50, 1949.

Marinacci, A. A.: The use of electromyography in the differential diagnosis of lumbar herniated disks, Bull. Los Angeles Neurol. Soc. 23:65-71, 1958.

Marinacci, A. A.: Myotonia of the lower axial musculature simulating lumbar spinal nerve root lesions, Bull. Los Angeles Neurol. Soc. 24:166-173, 1959.

Marinacci, A. A.: Electromyogram in the evaluation of lumbar herniated disc, Bull. Los Angeles Neurol. Soc. 30:47-62, 1965.

Marinacci, A. A., and Rand, C. W.: Total demyelinization of the peripheral nerves simulating surgical lumbar herniated disk, Bull. Los Angeles Neurol. Soc. 26:62-67, 1961.

Marr, J. T.: Gas in intervertebral discs, Amer. J. Roentgen. 70:804-809, 1953.

Marshall, W. J., and Schorstein, J.: Factors affecting the results of surgery for prolapsed lumber intervertebral disc, Scot. Med. J. 13:38-42, 1968.

Martin, J.: Diagnoses and treatment of herniation of intervertebral disc, Arizona Med. 4:29-32, 1947.

Martz, C. D.: Lumbar nuclear herniation and resulting physical impairment, J. Indiana Med. Ass. 48:33-37, 1955.

Masturzo, A.: Vertebral traction for treatment of sciatica, Rheumatism 11:62-67, 1955.

Mathews, J. A., and Yates, D. A.: Reduction of lumbar disc prolapse by manipulation, Brit. Med. J. 3:696-697, 1969.

Mayfield, F. H.: Herniated nucleus pulposus; protruded intervertebral discs, Mich. Med. 44:1206-1209, 1945.

McBride, E. D.: Herniated intervertebral disc, indications for morticed bone-block fusion, J. Okla. Med. Ass. 45:100-102, 1952.

McCaskin, F. B.: Pathologic alterations associated with induced inflammatory lesions of the intervertebral discs in dogs, an experimental study, Minneapolis, 1958 (thesis Univ. Minnesota).

McClintock, H. G.: Herniated lumbar disc a surgical emergency, Amer. Surg. 26:785-787, 1960.

McClure, C., Holland, H. C., and Woodhall, B.: Method for quantitative determination of hyaluronic acid in human intervertebral disk, Science 119:189, 1954.

McEachern, D. S.: Lumbar disc protrusion; useful sign. J. Neurosurg. 9:229-230, 1952.

McKee, G. K.: Traction-manipulation and plastic corsets in treatment of disc lesions of the lumbar spine, Lancet 1:472-475, 1956.

McKenzie, D.: Case of prolapsed intervertebral disc with ante-mortem and post-mortem findings, Aust. New Zeal. J. Surg. 16:219-224, 1947.

McNeur, J. C.: Tumours of proximal limb bones and hip simulating intervertebral disc lesions, Proc. Roy. Soc. Med. 46:351-352, 1953.

McRae, D. L.: Asymptomatic intervertebral disc protrusions, Acta Radiol. 46:9-27, 1956.

Mealey, J., Jr.: Fat emulsion as a cause of cloudy cerebrospinal fluid, J.A.M.A. 180:246-248, 1962.

Meirowsky, A. M., Scheibert, C. D., and First, T. D.: The syndrome of the herniated thoracic disc, Southern Med. J. 55:72-74, 1962.

Mendelsohn, R. A., and Sola, A.: Electromyography in herniated lumbar disks, Arch. Neurol. Psychiat. 79:142-145, 1958.

Mennell, J. M.: Backache, New Zeal. Med. J. 46:324-331, 1947.

Mennell, J. M.: Intervertebral disks and low backache, New Zeal. Med. J. 46:40-44, 1947.

Mennell, J. M.: Clinical evaluation of low-back pain and its treatment, Arch. Phys. Med. 36:78-87, 1955.

Mensor, M. C.: Non-operative treatment, including manipulation, for lumbar intervertebral disc syndrome, J. Bone Joint Surg. 37-A:925-936, 984, 1955.

Mensor, M. C.: Conservative treatment of intervertebral disc injuries, Calif. Med. 86:89-90, 1957.

Mensor: M. C.: Non-operative treatment, including manipulation, for lumbar intervertebral-disc syndrome, J. Bone Joint Surg. 47:1073-1074, 1965.

Meredith, J. M.: Familial sciatica due to herniated discs, Southern Surg. 14:258-263, 1948.

Meredith, J. M.: Intervertebral disc lesions, W. Virginia Med. J. 44:191-196, 1948.

Meredith, J. M.: The vagaries and peculiarities of studies with subarachnoid oil in cases of protruded disc: a plea for early

study with oil after negative or even positive surgical exploration for protrusion of
lumbar and cervical discs with persistent
postoperative symptoms, Southern Med. J.
52:322-329, 1959.

Michaelis, R., and Ashcroft, C.: Treatment
of lumbar disc protrusions by full range
movement, Physiotherapy **47:**184-186,
1961.

Michele, A. A., and Krueger, F. J.: Surgical
approach to vertebral body, J. Bone Joint
Surg. **31-A:**873-878, 1949.

Miller, D.: Follow-up study of 264 cases of
intervertebral disc lesion treated surgically,
Aust. New Zeal. J. Surg. **24:**63-65, 1954.

Miller, D.: Sciatica due to intervertebral
disc lesions; a personal review, Med. J.
Aust. **49:**621-624, 1962.

Miller, D., and Vanderfield, G.: Clinicopathological observations on lumbar intervertebral disk protrusion; account of 53 consecutive cases treated by operation at one
centre, Med. J. Aust. **2:**200-202, 1947.

Miller, R., McCollough, N. C., and Jewett,
E. L.: Early ambulation of low-fused back,
J. Florida Med. Ass. **36:**211-215, 1949.

Miller, W. A., and Ellis, K. W.: The use of
Pantopaque myelography in the diagnosis
of lumbar disc disease, J. Okla. Med. Ass.
62:23-29, 1969.

Millikan, C. H.: Problem of evaluating treatment of protruded lumbar intervertebral
disk; observations of results of conservative
and surgical treatment in 429 cases,
J.A.M.A. **155:**1141-1143, 1954.

Milone, F. P., Bianco, A. J., Jr., and Ivins,
J. C.: Infections of the intervertebral disk
in children, J.A.M.A. **181:**1029-1033, 1962.

Mitchell, P. E., Hendry, N. G., and Bille-
wicz, W. Z.: The chemical background of
intervertebral disc prolapse, J. Bone Joint
Surg. **43-B:**141-151, 1961.

Mixter, W. J.: Rupture of intervertebral disk;
short history of evolution as syndrome of
importance to surgeon, J.A.M.A. **140:**278-
282, 1949.

Mixter, W. J.: Pitfalls in surgery of ruptured
intervertebral disk, J. Florida Med. Ass.
39:159-167, 1952.

Mixter, W. J., and Barr, J. S.: Rupture of the
intervertebral disc with involvement of the
spinal canal, Clin. Orthop. **27:**3-8, 1963.

Moody, L.: Nursing care: patients with herniated discs, Canad. Nurse **61:**204-206,
1965.

Mooney, A. C.: Disc lesions in relation to
pain, Brit. J. Radiol. **18:**153-157, 1945.

Moore, A. T.: Unstable spine; discogenetic
syndrome treatment with self-locking prop
bone graft, J. Int. Coll. Surg. **8:**64-75, 1945;
correction **8:**179, 1945.

Moore, A. T., and Cook, W. C.: Lame back
with or without sciatica, J. S. Carolina
Med. Ass. **44:**41-42, 1948.

Moore, C. A., and Cohen, A.: Combined arterial, venous, and ureteral injury complicating lumbar disk surgery, Amer. J. Surg.
115:574-577, 1968.

Mori, M., and Ogawa, R.: Osteoplastic partial laminectomy for removing the lumber
disc herniation, Arch. Jap. Chir. **35:**873-
878, 1966.

Morrell, R. M.: Herniated lumbar intervertebral disc; cutaneous hyperalgesia as
an early sign, Milit. Med. **124:**257-269,
1959.

Morrissey, E. J.: Surgical lesions simulating
lumbar disc syndrome, Western J. Surg.
59:643-647, 1951.

Motley, L.: Neurogenic pain stimulating
visceral disease, Amer. J. Med. **4:**539-544,
1948.

Munro, D.: Diagnosis of posterior herniation
of lumbar intervertebral discs, New Eng.
J. Med. **232:**149-160, 1945.

Munro, D.: Lumbar and sacral compression
radiculitis: herniated lumbar disk syndrome, New Eng. J. Med. **254:**243-252,
1956.

Munslow, R. A., and Hinchey, J. J.: Protruded intervertebral disk syndrome; con-
servatism in management, Texas Med.
46:24-27, 1950.

Murphy, A. L.: Protruded lumbar intervertebral disc; toward its more exact
localization, Nova Scotia Med. Bull.
20:262-265, 1947; Manitoba Med. Rev.
28:9-10, 1948.

Murphy, J. P.: Lumbar intervertebral disc
protrusion contralateral to side of symptoms and signs; myleographic verification
in 2 cases, Amer. J. Roentgen. **61:**77-79,
1949.

Murphy, J. P.: Protrusion or rupture of
lumbar intervertebral disks; principal
cause of low back pain with sciatica, Med.
Ann. D. C. **24:**277-286, 1955.

Murray, A. R.: Lumbar intervertebral disk
lesion, Med. J. Aust. **2:**884-888, 1953.

Muscolo, D.: Semilogiá de la protusión del
disco intervertebral, Día Méd. **17:**122-124,
1945.

Nachemson, A.: Physical changes in the prolapsed disc, Lancet **1:**1150, 1959.

Nachemson, A.: Lumbar intradiscal pressure.
Experimental studies on postmortem material, Acta Orthop. Scand. supp 43:1-104,
1960.

Nachemson, A.: Oxyphenbutazone (Tanderil)
in surgery for herniated discs. A double
blind trial, Acta Orthop. Scand. **37:**267-
275, 1966.

Nachlas, I. W., chairman: Research Committee of the American Orthopaedic Association: End-result study of treatment of
herniated nucleus pulposus by excision

with fusion and without fusion, J. Bone Joint Surg. **34-A**:981-988, 1952.

Naiman, J. L., Donohue, W. L., and Prichard, J. S.: Fatal nucleus pulposus embolism of spinal cord after trauma, Neurology **11**:83-87, 1961.

Nathanson, M.: Paroxysmal phenomena resembling seizures, related to spinal cord and root pathology, case report, J. Mount Sinai Hosp. N. Y. **29**:147-151, 1962.

Naylor, A.: The biophysical and biochemical aspects of intervertebral disc herniation and degeneration, Ann. Roy. Coll. Surg. Eng. **31**:91-114, 1962.

Naylor, A., Happey, F., and MacRae, T.: Changes in human intervertebral disc with age: biophysical study, J. Amer. Geriat. Soc. **3**:964-973, 1955.

Naylor, A., and Horton, W. G.: Hydrophilic properties of nucleus pulposus of intervertebral disc, Rheumatism **11**:32-35, 1955.

Naylor, A., and Smare, D. L.: Fluid content of nucleus pulposus as factor in disc syndrome; preliminary report, Brit. Med. J. **2**:975-976, 1953.

Naylor, A., and Turner, R. L.: ACTH in treatment of lumbar disc prolapse, Proc. Roy. Soc. Med. **54**:282-284, 1961.

Neuwirth, E.: Management of sciatica by vertebral traction by means of mechanical table, Rheumatism **10**:12-17, 1954.

Neuwirth, E., Hilde, W., and Campbell, R.: Tables for vertebral elongation in treatment of sciatica, Arch. Phys. Med. **33**:455-460, 1952.

Noyes, M. B., and Hunter, J. A.: Evaluation of operative treatment of ruptured lumbar discs, J. Int. Coll. Surg. **16**:746-752, 1951.

O'Connell, J. E.: Clinical diagnosis of lumbar intervertebral disk protrusions with indications for their operative removal, Brit. Med. J. **1**:122-124, 1946.

O'Connell, J. E.: Indications for and results of excision of lumbar intervertebral disc protrusions; review of 500 cases; Hunterian lecture, Ann. Roy. Coll. Surg. Eng. **6**:403-412, 1950.

O'Connell, J. E.: Protrusions of lumbar intervertebral discs; clinical review based on 500 cases treated by excision of protrusion (Hunterian lecture), J. Bone Joint Surg. **33-B**:8-30, 1951.

O'Connell, J. E.: Involvement of spinal cord by intervertebral disk protrusions, Brit. J. Surg. **43**:225-247, 1955.

O'Connell, J. E.: Intervertebral disk protrusions in childhood and adolescence, Brit. J. Surg. **47**:611-616, 1960.

O'Connell, J. E.: Lumbar disc protrusions in pregnancy, J. Neurol. Neurosurg. Psychiat. **23**:138-141, 1960.

O'Connell, J. E.: The treatment of protru-

sions of the lumbar intervertebral discs, Physiotherapy **50**:294-296, 1964.

Odell, R. T., Conrad, M., and Key, J. A.: Removal of lumbar intervertebral disks; postoperative results, Amer. Acad. Orthop. Surg. Lect. **11**:126-129, 1954.

Odell, R. T., and Key, J. A.: Lumbar disk syndrome caused by malignant tumors of bone, J.A.M.A. **157**:213-216, 1955.

Odell, R. T., Ramsey, R. H., and Key, J. A.: Results after operative removal of intervertebral disks, Southern Med. J. **43**:759-765, 1950.

O'Donoghue, D. H.: Acute back injuries, Med. Rec. Ann. **49**:348-352, 1955.

Oldberg, E.: Protruded intervertebral disc, Mississippi Valley Med. J. **67**:8-13, 1945.

Oldberg, E.: Syndrome of protruded intervertebral disk, Med. Clin. N. Amer. **32**:1403-1413, 1948.

Oldberg, E.: Low back pain; neurosurgical viewpoint, Industr. Med. Surg. **18**:16-19, 1949.

Oliver, L.: Multiple lumbar disc protrusions, Proc. Roy. Soc. Med. **57**:329, 1964.

Orofino, C., Sherman, M. S., and Schechter, D.: Luschka's joint—a degenerative phenomenon, J. Bone Joint Surg. **42-A**:853-858, 1960.

Ovens, J. M., and Williams, H. G.: Intervertebral spine fusion with removal of herniated intervertebral disk, Amer. J. Surg. **70**:24-26, 1945.

Overton, L. M.: Lumbosacral arthrodesis: an evaluation of its present status, Amer. Surg. **25**:771-775, 1959.

Padula, R. D., and Keys, R. C.: Ruptured intervertebral disc; postoperative follow-up study, J. Int. Coll. Surg. **18**:92-97, 1952.

Pagni, C. A., Cassinari, V., and Bernasconi, V.: Meningocele spurius following hemilaminectomy in a case of lumbar discal hernia, J. Neurosurg. **18**:709-710, 1961.

Palazzo, F. A.: The ruptured disk versus the protruded disk, Southern Med. J. **53**:55-62, 1960.

Parrella, G. S., and Zovickian, A.: The ruptured intervertebral disc problem in the veteran, Surgery **27**:762-769, 1950.

Parrish, T. F.: Lumbar disk surgery in patients over 50 years of age, Southern Med. J. **55**:667-669, 1962.

Pasternak, S.: The patient with a ruptured disk, Amer. J. Nurs. **62**:77-80, 1962.

Paterson, J. E., and Gray, W.: Herniated nucleus pulposus: free fragment, Brit. J. Surg. **39**:509-513, 1952.

Peacher, W. G., and Robertson, R. C. L.: Pantopaque myelography; results, comparison of contrast media and spinal fluid reaction, J. Neurosurg. **2**:220-231, 1945.

Peacher, W. G., and Storrs, R. P.: The roentgen diagnosis of herniated disk with particular reference to diskography (nucleography), Amer. J. Roentgen. **76**:290-302, 1956.

Peacock, A.: Observations on pre-natal development of intervertebral disc in man, J. Anat. **85**:260-274, 1951.

Pearce, J.: The lumbar disc syndrome, Postgrad. Med. J. **45**:278-284, 1969.

Pearce, J., and Moll, J. M.: Conservative treatment and natural history of acute lumbar disc lesions, J. Neurol. Neurosurg. Psychiat. **30**:13-17, 1967.

Perey, O.: Contrast medium examination of intervertebral discs of lower lumbar spine, Acta Orthop. Scand. **20**:327-334, 1951.

Perl, J. I.: Transabdominal anterior discographic examination, J. Int. Coll. Surg. **22**:76-84, 1954.

Perlmutter, I., et al.: Gram-negative infection following herniated lumbar intervertebral disc excision, J. Florida Med. Ass. **57**:25-27, 1970.

Perrett, L.: Lumbar discography, J. Coll. Radiol. Aust. **6**:54-59, 1962.

Peterson, H. O.: Value of x-ray examination in diagnosis of ruptured intervertebral disc, Minn. Med. **29**:904, 1946.

Petrie, J. G.: Conservative management of lumbar disk protrusions, Postgrad. Med. **38**:654-657, 1965.

Pettit, G. D.: The surgical treatment of cervical disc protrusions in the dog, Cornell Vet. **50**:259-282, 1960.

Peyton, W. T., and Simmons, D. R.: Herniated intervertebral disk; analysis of 90 cases, Arch. Surg. **55**:271-287, 1947.

Piatt, A. D.: Varicosities of spinal canal veins in lumbar region simulating disc herniations, Ohio Med. J. **45**:979-982, 1949.

Pilgaard, S.: Discitis. Closed-space infection after lumbar discus prolapse operation, Acta Orthop. Scand. **40**:681, 1969.

Pilgaard, S.: Discitis (closed space infection) following removal of lumbar intervertebral disc, J. Bone Joint Surg. **51**:713-716, 1969.

Platt, H.: Backache-sciatica syndrome and intervertebral disc, Rheumatism **4**:218, 1948.

Poppen, J. L.: Herniated intervertebral disk; analysis of 400 verified cases, New Eng. J. Med. **232**:211-215, 1945.

Potter, J. M.: Protruded disk sciatica in services and its management, J. Roy. Army Med. Corps **89**:143-148, 1947.

Prader, A.: Die Entwicklung der Zwischenwirbelscheibe beim menschlichen Keimling, Acta Anat. **3**:115-152, 1947.

Pridie, K. H.: Sciatica as orthopaedic problem, Practitioner **155**:84-88, 1945.

Pringle, B.: An approach to intervertebral disc lesions, Trans. Ass. Industr. Med. Off. **5**:127-134, 1956.

Quade, R. H.: Treatment of backache; neuro-

surgical aspects, Wisconsin Med. J. **44**:979-983, 1945.

Raaf, J.: Some observations regarding 905 patients operated upon for protruded lumbar intervertebral disc, Amer. J. Surg. **97**:388-397, 1959.

Raaf, J.: Removal of protruded lumbar intervertebral discs, J. Neurosurg. **32**:604-611, 1970.

Raaf, J., and Berglund, G.: Results of operations for lumbar protruded intervertebral disc, J. Neurosurg. **6**:160-168, 1949.

Rabinovitch, R.: Diseases of the intervertebral disc and its surrounding tissues, Springfield, Ill., 1961, Charles C Thomas, Publisher.

Raines, J. R.: Intervertebral disc fissures (vacuum intervertebral disc), Amer. J. Roentgen. **70**:964-966, 1953.

Ramsay, D. B.: Simple traction apparatus for use in general practice, Practitioner **172**:572-574, 1954.

Ramsey, F. A.: Surgical correction of calcified lumbar intervertebral disk in a Dachshund—a case report, J. Amer. Vet. Med. Ass. **137**:540-543, 1960.

Ramsey, R. H.: Conservative treatment of intervertebral disk lesions, Amer. Acad. Orthop. Surg. Lect. **11**:118-120, 1954.

Rana, R. S.: Conservative and operative treatment of 240 lumbar disc lesions, Neurol. India **17**:76-81, 1969.

Rand, R. W.: A new intervertebral and special angled curette for lumbar disk surgery, Bull. Los Angeles Neurol. Soc. **23**:180-181, 1958.

Rand, R. W., and Crandall, P. H.: Surgical treatment of cervical osteoarthritis, Calif. Med. **91**:185-188, 1959.

Raney, A. A., and Raney, R. B.: Postspinal headache; etiology and prophylaxis, Western J. Surg. **55**:550-554, 1947.

Raney, R. B.: Progress in orthopedic surgery for 1944; conditions involving lower part of back, Arch. Surg. **52**:342-360, 1946.

Raney, R. B.: Progress in orthopedic surgery for 1945; conditions involving lower part of back, Arch. Surg. **55**:87-100, 1947.

Raney, R. B., and Raney, A. A.: Consideration of etiology in development of ruptured intervertebral disc, Calif. Med. **68**:65-69, 1948.

Rasmussen, J. H.: Protrusion of second lumbar disc; report of 5 cases encountered among 1376 lumbar disc protrusions verified by operation, Acta Psychiat. Neurol. Scand. supp. 108:339-346, 1956.

Ray, B. S.: Differential diagnosis between ruptured lumbar intervertebral disk and certain diseases of spinal and peripheral nervous systems, Surg. Clin. N. Amer. **26**:272-281, 1946.

Re, C.: Notes on surgical technique and instrumental equipment in the operative treatment of discal lumbosciatalgia, Panminerva Med. 1:189-194, 1959.

Rechtman, A. M., Hermel, M. B., Albert, S. M., and Boreadis, A. G.: Calcification of intervertebral disk: disappearing, dormant and silent, Clin. Orthop., no. 7, 218-231, 1956.

Rees, S. E., and Donley, C. E.: Accuracy of Pantopaque studies in diagnosis of herniated intervertebral disc, Northwest. Med. 48:180-182, 1949.

Reynolds, F. C.: Intervertebral disk: surgical technique, Amer. Acad. Orthop. Surg. Lect. 11:121-125, 1954.

Reynolds, F. C., McGinnis, A. E., and Morgan, H. C.: Surgery in the treatment of low-back pain and sciatica; a follow-up study, J. Bone Joint Surg. 41-A:223-235, 1959.

Rhydderch, A. I.: Second thoughts on surgery of the lumbar disc, Western J. Surg. 72:139-141, 1964.

Rix, R. R.: Intraspinal myelography and herniated disc in lumbar spine, J. Maine Med. Ass. 36:169-173, 1945.

Roberts, R. A.: Chronic structural low backache due to low-back structural derangement, London, 1947, H. K. Lewis & Co., Ltd.

Roberts, R. A.: Deossification in lumbar transverse process, Brit. J. Radiol. 22:540-543, 1949.

Robertson, R. C. L.: Ruptured intervertebral disc in industry, Southern Med. J. 42:891-895, 1949.

Robertson, R. C. L., and Peacher, W. G.: Herniation of nucleus pulposus; refinement in operative technique, Surgery 18:768-772, 1945.

Robinson, R. G.: Massive protrusions of lumbar disks, Brit. J. Surg. 52:858-865, 1965.

Roelsgaard, M.: Prolapse of lumbar intervertebral disk and chondrosarcoma of pelvis in same patient, Nord. Med. 41:1105-1106, 1949.

Rogers, L.: Sciatica, J. Roy. Nav. Med. Serv. 32:209-211, 1946.

Rogers, L.: Intervertebral discs and sciatica, J. Roy. Nav. Med. Serv. 36:125-131, 1950.

Rombold, C.: Sciatica secondary to retropulsed intervertebral discs, J. Kansas Med. Soc. 46:253-256, 1945.

Rombold, C.: Intervertebral disc syndrome, GP 3:67-69, 1951.

Rombold, C.: Role of intervertebral disc in backache, J. Kansas Med. Soc. 54:373-377, 1953.

Rombold, C., Anderson, H. O., and Marsh, H. O.: Report on 116 cases of intervertebral discs, J. Kansas Med. Soc. 49:453-455, 1948.

Rose, G. K.: Backache and disc, Lancet 1:1143-1149, 1954.

Rose, G. K.: Prolapsed intervertebral disc, Med. Illus. 9:219-232, 1955.

Roseman, E.: Pain associated with protruded intervertebral disks, Med. Clin. N. Amer. 42:1567-1588, 1958.

Rosomoff, H. L., Johnston, J. D., Gallo, A. E., Givens, F., and Kuehn, C. A.: Routine cystometry in evaluation of lumbar disk syndromes, Surg. Forum 13:442-443, 1962.

Ross, P., and Jelsma, F.: Postoperative analysis of 366 consecutive cases of herniated lumbar discs, Amer. J. Surg. 84:657-662, 1952.

Rothenberg, S. F., Mendelsohn, H. A., and Putnam, T. J.: Effect of leg traction on ruptured intervertebral discs, Surg. Gynec. Obstet. 96:564-566, 1953.

Rövig, G.: Rupture of lumbar discs with intraspinal protrusion of nucleus pulposus. Clinical study, Acta Chir. Scand. 99:175-180, 1949.

Rowbotham, G. F., and Whalley, N.: Low backache, sciatic pain and herniated nucleus pulposus, Practitioner 160:212-220, 1948.

Rubinstein, B. M., Stern, W. Z., and Jacobson, H. G.: Block of the spinal cord caused by herniated disk, Amer. J. Roentgen. 81:1011-1020, 1959.

Rugtveit, A.: Juvenile lumbar disc herniations, Acta Orthop. Scand. 37:348-356, 1966.

Runyon, S. S.: A correlation of diagnostic studies with operative findings on the lumbar intervertebral disks, J. Amer. Osteopath. Ass. 60:750-752, 1961.

Sallis, J. G.: Re-exploration of the lumbar intervertebral disc, S. Afr. Med. J. 38:895-896, 1964.

Sallis, J. G., and Smith, R. G.: Vertebral venography in the diagnosis of prolapsed intervertebral disc, Proc. Roy. Soc. Med. 55:502-504, 1962.

Samuel, E.: Vacuum intervertebral discs, Brit. J. Radiol. 21:337-339, 1948.

Sandström, C.: Calcifications of intervertebral discs and relationship between various types of calcifications in soft tissues of body, Acta Radiol. 36:217-233, 1951.

Sayle-Creer, W. S.: Degenerative changes in intervertebral discs, Rheumatism 12:2-11, 1956.

Scheman, L., and Fraerman, S. H.: An effective laminotomy rest, J. Bone Joint Surg. 39-A:670-671, 1957.

Scherbel, A. L., and Gardner, W. J.: Infections involving the intervertebral disks. Diagnosis and management, J.A.M.A. 174:370-374, 1960.

Schlesinger, E. B., and Stinchfield, F. E.:

Use of myanesin as prognostic test in treatment of acute low back disorders, Trans. Amer. Neurol. Ass. **75:**201-205, 1950.

Schlesinger, E. B., and Stinchfield, F. E.: Use of muscle relaxants as aid in diagnosis and therapy of acute low-back disorders, J. Bone Joint Surg. **33-A:**480-484, 501, 504, 1951.

Schlesinger, E. B., and Taveras, J. M.: Factors in production of "cauda equina" syndromes in lumbar discs, Trans. Amer. Neurol. Ass. **78:**263-265, 1953.

Schneider, R. C.: Chronic neurological sequelae of acute trauma to the spine and spinal cord. II. The syndrome of chronic anterior spinal cord injury or compression; herniated intervertebral discs, J. Bone Joint Surg. **41-A:**449-456, 1959.

Schnitker, M. T., and Booth, G. T.: Pantopaque myelography for protruded discs of lumbar spine, Radiology **45:**370-376, 1945.

Schnitker, M. T., and Curtzwiler, F. C.: Hypertrophic osteosclerosis (bony spur) of the lumbar spine; producing the syndrome of protruded intervertebral disc with sciatic pain, J. Neurosurg. **14:**121-128, 1957.

Schreiber, F., and Rosenthal, H.: Paraplegia from ruptured lumbar discs in achondroplastic dwarfs, J. Neurosurg. **9:**648-651, 1952.

Schwartz, H. G.: Ruptured cervical intervertebral disks, Postgrad. Med. **11:**501-506, 1952.

Schweitzer, E. H.: Manipulation of lumbosacral joint, Ohio Med. J. **47:**930-932, 1951.

Scott, J. C.: Stress factor in disc syndrome, J. Bone Joint Surg. **37:**107-111, 1955.

Scougall, S. H.: The conservative treatment of the injured back, Med. J. Aust. **2:**566-570, 1949.

Scoville, W. B., Moretz, W. H., and Hankins, W. D.: Discrepancies in myelography; statistical survey of 200 operative cases undergoing Pantopaque myelography, Surg. Gynec. Obstet. **86:**559-564, 1948.

Scuderi, C.: Herniated lumbar intervertebral disks; an eight-year survey, Amer. J. Surg. **91:**481-483, 1956.

Scuderi, C., and Khedroo, F.: Herniation of intervertebral disc; diagnosis, treatment and résumé of follow-up study, J. Int. Coll. Surg. **23:**194-203, 1955.

Seeley, S. F., Hughes, C. W., and Jahnke, E. J., Jr.: Major vessel damage in lumbar disc operation, Surgery **35:**421-429, 1954.

Sell, L. S.: Misdiagnosis and mismanagement of early intervertebral disc lesions, J.A.M.A. **150:**987-990, 1952.

Semmes, R. E.: Ruptured lumbar intervertebral discs: their recognition and surgical relief, Clin. Neurosurg. **8:**78-92, 1962.

Semmes, R. E., and Murphey, F.: Symposium on neurological surgery; ruptured intervertebral disks: cervical, thoracic and lumbar, lateral and central, Surg. Clin. N. Amer. **34:**1095-1111, 1954.

Senseman, L. A., Hamlin, H., and Umstead, H.: Ruptured intervertebral discs—diagnosis and treatment, Rhode Island Med. J. **32:**378-380, 1949.

Serensen, H. R.: Guide for use in x-raying lumbar column in lumbo-inguinal projection, Acta Orthop. Scand. **23:**87-89, 1953.

Sewell, R. L.: Ruptured intervertebral disc, Texas Med. **41:**357-369, 1945.

Shannon, P. W., and Terhune, S. R.: Low back problem, Amer. Surg. **17:**1106-1112, 1951.

Sheldon, K. W.: False fear of disc surgery, Nebraska Med. J. **34:**326-329, 1949.

Shenkin, H. A., and Haft, H.: Foraminotomy in the surgical treatment of herniated lumbar disks, Surgery **60:**274-279, 1966.

Shephard, R. H.: Diagnosis and prognosis of cauda equina syndrome produced by protrusion of lumbar disk, Brit. Med. J. **2:**1434-1449, 1959.

Sherbok, B. C.: A maneuver of help in diagnosis of ruptured disk, Arch. Surg. **76:**986-987, 1958.

Sherman, I. J., and Cook, W. H.: Diagnostic features of herniated lumbar disc (survey of 1000 conservative surgically treated cases), Conn. Med. **26:**475-478, 1962.

Shinners, B. M., and Hamby, W. B.: Protruded lumbar intervertebral discs; results following surgical and non-surgical therapy, J. Neurosurg. **6:**450-457, 1949.

Shroyer, R. N., Fortson, C. H., and Theodotou, C. B.: Delayed neurological sequelae of a retained foreign body (lead bullet) in the intervertebral disc space, J. Bone Joint Surg. **42-A:**595-599, 1960.

Shumacker, H. B., Jr., King, H., and Campbell, R.: Vascular complications from disc operations, J. Trauma **1:**177-185, 1961.

Shutkin, N. M.: Syndrome of degenerated intervertebral disc, Amer. J. Surg. **84:**162-171, 1952.

Siehl, D.: Manipulation of the spine under general anesthesia, J. Amer. Osteopath. Ass. **62:**881-887, 1963.

Simon, S. D., Silver, C. M., and Litchman, H. H.: Lumbar disk surgery in the elderly (over the age of 60), Clin. Orthop. **41:**157-162, 1965.

Siris, J. H.: Some problems of traumatic causal relationship in development of lumbar disk hernia, New York J. Med. **52:**717-720, 1952.

Siris, J. H.: Preoperative localization of intervertebral disk hernias and other cord-compressing lesions, New York J. Med. **53:**1677-1681, 1953.

Siris, J. H., and Miller, M. L.: Spinal anesthesia in lumbar disc surgery, Anesth. Analg. **31:**208-210, 1952.

Skobowytsh-Okolot, B.: "Posterior apophysis" in L. IV—the cause of neuradicular disturbance, Acta Orthop. Scand. **32**:341-351, 1962.

Skouron, M.: Improved retractor for intervertebral-disc surgery, J. Bone Joint Surg. **29**:247, 1947.

Slater, R. A., Pineda, A., and Porter, R. W.: Intradural herniation of lumbar intervertebral discs, Arch. Surg. **90**:266-269, 1965.

Slemmer, R. E.: Diagnosis of herniation of lumbar intervertebral disc (nucleus pulposus), Ohio Med. J. **45**:345-348, 1949.

Slim, D.: Sustained traction for lumbar spinal lesions, Physiotherapy **44**:282-286, 1958.

Smith, B. H.: Intervertebral disc in forensic medicine, Industr. Med. Surg. **24**:36-40, 1955.

Smith, F. P.: Transvertebral rupture of intervertebral disc., J. Neurosurg. **19**:594-598, 1962.

Smith, J. W., and Walmsley, R.: Experimental incision of intervertebral disc, J. Bone Joint Surg. **33-B**:612-625, 1951.

Smith, L., and Brown, J. E.: Treatment of lumbar intervertebral disc lesions by direct injection of chymopapain, J. Bone Joint Surg. **49**:502-519, 1967.

Smith, R. N.: Anatomical factors influencing disc protrusion in dog and man, Proc. Roy. Soc. Med. **51**:571-573, 1958.

Smolik, E. A., and Nash, F. P.: Lumbar spinal arachnoiditis; complication of intervertebral disc operation, Ann. Surg. **133**:490-495, 1951.

Smyth, M. J., and Wright, V.: Sciatica and the intervertebral disc; an experimental study, J. Bone Joint Surg. **40-A**:1401-1418, 1958.

Sneider, S. E., Winslow, O. P., Jr., and Pryor, T. H.: Cervical diskography: is it relevant? J.A.M.A. **185**:163-165, 1963.

Snellman, A.: Pathogenesis of disk prolapse in lumbar region of spine and question of compensation for resulting morbid condition, Nord. Med. (Duodecim) **27**:1517-1523, 1945.

Söderberg, L., and Andrèn, L.: Disc degeneration and lumbago-ischias, Acta Orthop. Scand. **25**:137-148, 1955.

Söderberg, L., and Sjoberg, S.: On operated herniated lumbar discs, Acta Orthop. Scand. **31**:146-151, 1961.

Soll, R. W.: Herniated intervertebral disc, Minnesota Med. **48**:1507-1513, 1965.

Song, J. U., and Ransohoff, J.: Surgical lesions of spine and spinal cord stimulating disk syndrome, New York J. Med. **62**:556-559, 1962.

Soule, A. B., Jr., Gross, S. W., and Irving, J. G.: Myelography by use of Pantopaque in diagnosis of herniations of intervertebral discs, Amer. J. Roentgen. **53**:319-340, 1945.

Spadea, S., and Hamlin, H.: Interspinous fusion for treatment of herniated inter-

vertebral discs utilizing lumbar spinous process as bone graft, Ann. Surg. **136**:982-986, 1952.

Spanos, N. C., and Andrew, J.: Intermittent claudication and lateral lumbar disc protrusions, J. Neurol. Neurosurg. Psychiat. **29**:273-277, 1966.

Speed, J. S., Stewart, M. J., and Trout, P. C.: Ruptured intervertebral discs; pathologic, diagnostic and therapeutic considerations, Southern Surg. **13**:645-652, 1947.

Speigel, I. J.: Herniation of the intervertebral disc. A systematized technique for treatment of lumbo-sacral and low lumbar lesions, Illinois Med. J. **89**:188-196, 1946.

Sperl, M. P., Jr., Nichols, D. R., Martin, W. J., MacCarty, C. S., and Henderson, E. D.: Some observations on the prophylactic use of procaine-penicillin in operations for protruded intervertebral disk with spinal fusion, J. Neurosurg. **13**:444-448, 1956.

Spira, E.: Problem of hernia disci intervertebralis; results of conservative therapy, Acta Med. Orient. **4**:109-122, 1945.

Spittell, J. A., Jr., Palumbo, P. J., Love, J. G., and Ellis, F. H., Jr.: Arteriovenous fistula complicating lumbar-disk surgery, New Eng. J. Med. **268**:1162-1165, 1963.

Spurling, R. G., and Grantham, E. G.: Ruptured intervertebral discs in lower lumbar regions, Amer. J. Surg. **75**:140-158, 1948.

Spurling, R. G., and Grantham, E. G.: End-results of surgery for ruptured lumbar intervertebral discs; follow-up study of 327 cases, J. Neurosurg. **6**:57-64, 1949.

Stafford, D. E.: Modern concepts of neurosurgical treatment of herniated nucleus pulposus, Northwest. Med. **46**:358-360, 1947.

Stanton, G. A.: Low back pain, Practitioner **190**:517-523, 1963.

Stein, R. O.: Anterior spine fusion—case report, Bull. Hosp. Joint Dis. **13**:322-327, 1952.

Steinberg, I., Glenn, F., Carver, S. T., and Lukas, D. S.: Angiographic and hemodynamic studies of a postlaminectomy iliac arterial interior vena canal fistula. Cure by incision and suture of the lesion, Amer. J. Med. **31**:310-317, 1961.

Steindler, A.: Analysis and differentiation of low-back pain in relation to the disc factor, J. Bone Joint Surg. **29**:455-460, 1947.

Steindler, A.: Pathomechanics of sacrolumbar junction, Instruct. Lect. Amer. Acad. Orthop. Surg. **12**:177-188, 1955.

Steiness, I.: Biothesiometry in the diagnosis of lumbar disk protrusion, Neurology **8**:793-795, 1958.

Stellar, S.: Neurosurgical aspects of low back pain, Compensat. Med. **6**:19-24, 1954.

Stender, A.: Treatment of sciatica (including that caused from herniated discs) by presacral injection of novocaine, J. Neuropath. Clin. Neurol. **1:**301-308, 1951.

Stenström, R.: Widening of root defect in lumbar myelogram by Abrodil, Acta Radiol. **29:**303-306, 1948.

Stern, M. B., and Mendelsohn, H. A.: Laminectomy for herniated intervertebral disc, Calif. Med. **91:**65-67, 1959.

Stern, W. E.: Lumbar intervertebral disc disease syndrome; clinical correlation of 175 cases, Western J. Surg. **63:**647-653, 1955.

Stern, W. E., and Crandall, P. H.: Inflammatory intervertebral disc disease as a complication of the operative treatment of lumbar herniations, J. Neurosurg. **16:**261-276, 1959.

Stewart, D. Y.: Anterior approach to degenerative disk disease of the cervical spine, New York J. Med. **61:**3085-3096, 1961.

Stewart, D. Y.: The anterior disk excision and interbody fusion approach to the problem of degenerative disk disease of the lower lumbar spinal segments, New York J. Med. **61:**3252-3262, 1961.

Stinchfield, F. E., and Cruess, R. L.: Indications for spine fusion in conjunction with removal of herniated nucleus pulposus, Instruct. Lect. Amer. Acad. Orthop. Surg. **18:**41-45, 1961.

Stinchfield, F. E., and Sinton, W. A.: Criteria for spine fusion with use of "H" bone graft following disc removal; results in 100 cases, Arch. Surg. **65:**542-550, 1952.

Stinchfield, F. E., and Sinton, W. A.: Clinical significance of transitional lumbosacral vertebra; relationship to back pain, disc disease, and sciatica, J.A.M.A. **157:**1107-1109, 1955.

Stoddard, A.: Manipulative procedures in treatment of intervertebral disc lesions, Brit. J. Phys. Med. **14:**101-106, 1951.

Storino, H. E., Siekert, R. G., and MacCarty, C. S.: Protrusion of lumbar disks causing marked bilateral weakness of the legs, Minn. Med. **41:**687-690, 1958.

Storck, H.: Die Lumbo-sakro-ischiopathie, Arch. Phys. Ther. **3:**121-141, 1951.

Stuck, R. M.: Surgical removal of ruptured cervical intervertebral discs, Rocky Mountain Med. J. **57:**36-39, 1960.

Stuck, R. M.: Results of anterior excision of ruptured cervical discs, Amer. Surg. **27:**469-470, 1961.

Stuck, R. M.: Anterior cervical disc excision and fusion; report of 200 consecutive cases, Rocky Mountain Med. J. **60:**25-30, 1963.

Stuck, R. M., Hall, R. F., and Fralick, E. H.: Anterior excision of ruptured cervical intervertebral disc and interbody fusion (Cloward), Amer. Surg. **26:**50-56, 1960.

Sullivan, C. R.: Diagnosis and treatment of pyogenic infections of the intervertebral disk, Surg. Clin. N. Amer. **41:**1077-1086, 1961.

Svaar, O.: Experiences in surgical treatment of lumbar disk herniation, Acta Chir. Scand. **109:**97-105, 1955.

Svien, H. J., Adson, A. W., and Dodge, H. W., Jr.: Lumbar extradural hematoma; report of case simulating protruded disk syndrome, J. Neurosurg. **7:**587-588, 1950.

Swett, P. P.: Note on sciatica, backache and intervertebral discs, Conn. Med. **9:**701-702, 1945.

Sylven, B., Paulson, S. C., Hirsch, C., and Snellman, O.: Biophysical and physiological investigations on cartilage and other mesenchymal tissues; ultrastructure of bovine and human nuclei pulposi, J. Bone Joint Surg. **33-A:**333-340, 1951.

Symonds, C.: Symptomatology and treatment of displaced intervertebral discs, Trans. Med. Soc. London (1946-1948) **65:**23-38, 1949.

Taher, Y., Sorour, O., el Shafie, I., et al.: Cauda equina lesion due to prolapsed lumbar intervertebral discs, J. Egypt. Med. Ass. **49:**336-346, 1966.

Takahashi, Y.: An autopsy case of the anterior spinal artery syndrome, Acta Path. Jap. **9** (supp.):905-912, 1959.

Tanz, S. S.: To-and-fro motion range at fourth and fifth lumbar interspaces, J. Mount Sinai Hosp. N. Y. **16:**303-307, 1950.

Taylor, A. R., Gleadhill, C. A., Bilsland, W. L., and Murphy, P. F.: Posture and anesthesia for spinal operations with special reference to intervertebral disc surgery, Brit. J. Anaesth. **28:**213-219, 1956.

Taylor, H., and Williams, E.: Arteriovenous fistula following disc surgery, Brit. J. Surg. **50:**47-50, 1962.

Taylor, T. K.: Treatment of lumbar disk prolapse, GP **32:**141-148, 1965.

Thibodeau, A. A.: Closed space infection following removal of lumbar intervertebral disc, J. Bone Joint Surg. **50:**400-410, 1968; Clin. Neurosurg. **14:**337-360, 1966.

Thomson, J. L.: Diagnosis and treatment of herniated nucleus pulposus, Virginia Med. Monthly **74:**365-368, 1947.

Titrud, L. A., Ritchie, W. P., and French, L. A.: Treatment of patients having prolapsed intervertebral discs in U. S. Army hospital overseas, Med. Bull. Mediterranean Theat. Op. **3:**251-256, 1945.

Törmä, T.: Postoperative recurrence of lumbar disc herniation, Acta Chir. Scand. **103:**213-221, 1952.

Toumey, J. W.: Intervertebral disk protrusion; selection of cases—types of surgery—after-care, Surg. Clin. N. Amer. **30:**941-943, 1950.

Tovi, D., and Strang, R. R.: Thoracic intervertebral disk protrusions, Acta Chir. Scand. supp. 267:1-41, 1960.

Troland, C. E.: Low back pain with sciatica; importance of ruptured intervertebral disc, Southern Med. Surg. 111:201, 203, 1949.

Troup, J. D.: Diagnosis of disc lesions, Lancet 2:642-643, 1961.

Troup, J. D.: Disc lesions, J. Coll. Gen. Pract. 4:101-105, 1961.

Troup, J. D.: The significance of disc lesions, Lancet 2:43-45, 1961.

Troup, J. D.: The anatomy and clinical pathology of the intervertebral disk, J. Amer. Osteopathy Ass. 62:193-196, 1962.

Trowbridge, W. V., and French, J. D.: "False positive" lumbar myelogram, Neurology 4:339-344, 1954.

Trumble, H. C.: Some aspects of diagnosis and treatment of prolapsed intervertebral discs, Aust. New Zeal. J. Surg. 15:159-165, 1946.

Turek, S. L.: Failure of disc operations; causes and technic of operation, Amer. J. Surg. 87:241-246, 1954.

Turnbull, F.: Postoperative inflammatory disease of lumbar discs, J. Neurosurg. 10:469-473, 1953.

Turner, V.: The rationale of the non-operative management of lesions of the lumbar intervertebral disc, Quart. Bull. Northw. Univ. Med. Sch. 33:279-281, 1959.

Tyrrell, J. B.: Diagnosis of herniation of lumbar disks, J.A.M.A. 128:540, 1945.

Uihlein, A., and Baker, H. L.: Centrally herniated intervertebral disk, Minn. Med. 51:1229-1233, 1968.

Unander-Scharin, L.: Results of lumbar osteosynthesis in disk degeneration, Nord. Med. 36:2205-2206, 1947.

Unander-Scharin, L.: On low-back pain, with special reference to value of operative treatment with fusion; clinical and experimental study, Acta Orthop. Scand. supp. 5:1-221, 1950.

Urist, M. R.: Processed cortical bone for internal fixation in lumbosacral arthrodesis. An application of the distraction-impaction principle to increase the intervertebral canal and disc spaces, Acta Orthop. Scand. 32:357-358, 1962.

Valobra, G.: Ultrasonic therapy for prolapsed intervertebral discs, Brit. J. Phys. Med. 17:109-110, 1954.

Van Allen, M. W.: Herniated lumbar intervertebral discs: diagnosis and management, Mississippi Valley Med. J. 76:130-133, 1954.

Van Driest, J. J., and Maxwell, H. P.: Central lumbar disk simulating cauda equina tumor occurring in 12-year-old boy with dyschondroplasia, Wisconsin Med. J. 51:374-375, 1952.

van Went, J. M.: Prolapsed intervertebral discs treated with ultrasonic waves, Brit. J. Phys. Med. 15:120-121, 1952.

Ver Brugghen, A.: Massive extrusions of lumbar intervertebral discs, Surg. Gynec. Obstet. 81:269-277, 1945.

Vernon, S.: Discogenic disease, backache and connective tissue function, J. Amer. Geriat. Soc. 8:195-199, 1960.

Villafane Lastra, T. de, and Griggs, J. F.: Brucellosis as a cause of herniated disk and spondylitis, Industr. Med. Surg. 26:122-129, 1957.

Virgin, W. J.: Experimental investigations into physical properties of intervertebral discs, J. Bone Joint Surg. 33-B:607-611, 1951.

Visser, S. L.: The significance of the Hoffmann reflex in the EMG examination of patients with herniation of the nucleus pulposus, Psychiat. Neurol. Neurochir. 68:300-305, 1965.

Voris, H. C.: Protrusion of intervertebral disk, Med. Clin. N. Amer. 29:111-125, 1945.

Voris, H. C.: Sudden extrusion of intervertebral disk, Dis. Nerv. Syst. 6:80-82, 1945.

Voris, H. C.: End results of "disc operations" in industry, J. Int. Coll. Surg. 21:198-204, 1954.

Walchef, L. S.: Traction brace; new traction method in conservative treatment of intervertebral disc lesions, Surgery 35:758-761, 1954.

Walk, L.: Diagnostic lumbar disc puncture; clinical review and analysis of 67 cases, Arch. Surg. 66:232-243, 1953.

Walk, L.: Lumbar diskography and its clinical evaluation, Bibl. Radiol. 3:1-135, 1962.

Walker, C. S.: Calcification of intervertebral discs in children, J. Bone Joint Surg. 36-B:601-605, 1954.

Walker, E.: Intervertebral disc lesions; general discussion and consideration of treatment in military service, Southern Med. J. 38:832-834, 1945.

Walker, E.: Rehabilitation of patients with ruptured intervertebral disks for heavy labor (new surgical approach), Southern Med. J. 49:1160-1163, 1956.

Walker, E., Miles, F. C., and Simpson, J. R.: Back disability 1930-1955, Amer. Surg. 21:1112-1120, 1955.

Walker, H. R.: Extradural osseous lesions simulating the disk syndrome, J.A.M.A. 172:691-694, 1960.

Walker, J. C.: Discography in the study and investigation of low back pain, Western J. Surg. 68:240-243, 1960.

Walmsley, R.: The development and growth of intervertebral disc (Sir John Struthers lecture), Edinburgh Med. J. 60:341-364, 1953.

Wanger, W. F., and Jewell, F. C.: Vacuum phenomenon in lumbosacral disc, Mich. Med. **52**:989-991, 1953.

Wardle, E. N.: Herniation of lumbar intervertebral disc and relationship to outer diseases of spine, Rheumatism **6**:143-148, 1950.

Wardy, R. C.: Herniated intervertebral lumbar disc. Current concepts in diagnosis and management, Texas Med. **61**:482-487, 1965.

Watson, R., and Shuffield, J. F.: Diagnostic aspects of ruptured intervertebral disks, J. Arkansas Med. Soc. **43**:212-215, 1947.

Waugh, O. S., Cameron, H. F., Scarrow, H. G., and Howarth, J. C.: Follow-up on lumbar disc lesions, Canad. Med. Ass. J. **61**:607-611, 1949.

Weaver, S. W.: Low back pain versus the intervertebral disc syndrome, Western J. Surg. **65**:19-24, 1957.

Webb, J. H., Svien, H. J., and Kennedy, R. L. J.: Protruded lumbar intervertebral disks in children, J.A.M.A. **154**:1153-1154, 1954.

Webster, F. S.: Myelography and intervertebral disc lesions of low back, Nebraska Med. J. **36**:386-390, 1951.

Webster, F. S., and Smiley, D. P.: End result study of a series of operations for herniated intervertebral lumbar discs, Amer. J. Surg. **99**:27-32, 1960.

Weiss, R. M.: Anterior removal of cervical intervertebral disk with interbody fusion, New York J. Med. **63**:86-91, 1963.

Weiss, S. R., and Raskind, R.: The teen-age "lumbar disk syndrome," Int. Surg. **49**:528-533, 1968.

Werden, D. H.: Intervertebral disc lesions; surgical treatment, end results, disability ratings and cost in industrial accident injuries, Calif. Med. **86**:84-88, 1957.

West, E. F.: Indications for operation on injured back, Med. J. Aust. **2**:314-315, 1949.

Wetzel, N., Arieff, A., and Tuncbay, E.: Retroperitoneal, lumbar, and pelvic malignancies simulating the "disc syndrome," Arch. Surg. **86**:1069-1071, 1963.

Whitcomb, B. B.: Symposium on problems in postwar medicine; rupture of intervertebral disk, Med. Clin. N. Amer. **30**:431-444, 1946.

White, J. C.: Results in surgical treatment of herniated lumbar intervertebral discs: investigation of the late results in subjects with and without supplementary spinal fusion—a preliminary report, Clin. Neurosurg. **13**:42-54, 1965.

White, J. C., and Peterson, T. H.: Lumbar herniations of intervertebral disks; value of surgical removal for naval personnel, Occup. Med. **1**:145-159, 1946.

White, J. W.: Conservative nonoperative treatment of lumbar disk lesions, Postgrad. Med. **16**:488-491, 1954.

Wiberg, G.: Back pain in relation to nerve supply of intervertebral disc, Acta Orthop. Scand. **19**:211-221, 1949.

Wieltberger, B. R., and Abbott, K. H.: Dowel intervertebral body fusion as used in lumbar disc therapy, J. Int. Coll. Surg. **29**:204-214, 1958.

Wiig, N.: The preoperative clinical diagnosis of lumbar disc prolapse; its reliability and practical applicability. A clinical study based on a series of 100 cases operated upon without preceding myelography, Acta Chir. Scand. supp. 295:1-100, 1962.

Williams, A. J., and Fullenlove, T.: Herniation of intervertebral discs; an evaluation of the indirect signs, Calif. Med. **83**:433-434, 1955.

Wilson, C. D.: Diagnosis and treatment of protruded lumbar intervertebral disks, Texas Med. **44**:445-449, 1948.

Wilson, D. H., and MacCarty, W. C.: Discography: its role in the diagnosis of lumbar disc protrusions, J. Neurosurg. **31**:520-523, 1969.

Wilson, D. M.: Prolapsed intervertebral disc and war pensioner, New Zeal. Med. J. **47**:322-337, 1948.

Wilson, J. C., Jr.: Degenerative arthritis of lumbar intervertebral joints. A clinical study, Amer. J. Surg. **100**:313-322, 1960.

Wilson, J. N.: Prolapsed intervertebral disk after lumbar puncture, Brit. Med. J. **2**:1334-1335, 1949.

Wilson, J. N., and Ilfield, F. W.: Manipulation of herniated intervertebral disc, Amer. J. Surg. **83**:173-175, 1952.

Wilson, P. D.: Low back pain and sciatica due to lesions of the lumbar discs. A study of results of surgical treatment, Rhode Island Med. J. **43**:167-173, 1960.

Wilson, P. J.: Cauda equina compression due to intrathecal herniation of an intervertebral disk: a case report, Brit. J. Surg. **49**:423-426, 1962.

Wilson, R. H.: Herniated intervertebral disks; time and cast analysis of 100 cases, Industr. Med. Surg. **20**:12-14, 1951.

Wiltberger, B. R.: Prefit dowel intervertebral body fusion as used in lumbar disc therapy; preliminary report, Amer. J. Surg. **86**:723-727, 1953.

Winkler, H., and Powers, J. A.: Meningocele following hemilaminectomy; report of 2 cases, N. Carolina Med. J. **11**:292-294, 1950.

Wise, B. L.: Disturbances of vibratory sense (pallesthesia) associated with nerve root compression due to herniated nucleus pulposus, Arch. Neurol. Psychiat. **68**:377-379, 1952.

Wise, C. S.: Herniation of the lumbar intervertebral disc, Rheumatism **17**:74-80, 1961.

Wise, C. S., and Adrizzone, J.: Electromyography in intervertebral disc protrusions, Arch. Phys. Med. 35:442-446, 1954.

Wise, C. S., and Rizzoli, H. V.: Herniation of the lumbar intervertebral disc, Bull. Rheum. Dis. 10:219-222, 1960.

Wolkin, J., Sachs, M. D., and Hoke, G. H.: Comparative studies of discography and myelography, Radiology 64:704-712, 1955.

Wolman, L.: Cramp in cases of prolapsed intervertebral disc, J. Neurol. Neurosurg. Psychiat. 12:251-257, 1949.

Woodhall, B., and Hayes, G. J.: Well-leg-raising test of Fajersztajn in diagnosis of ruptured lumbar intervertebral disc, J. Bone Joint Surg. 32-A:786-792, 1950.

Woolsey, R. D.: Herniation of the nucleus pulposus: experience in 600 cases and presentation of an apparently successful attempt to reduce the necessity for reoperation, J. Florida Med. Ass. 46:965-969, 1960.

Woolsey, R. D., and Coldwater, K. B.: Surgical treatment of intervertebral disk lesions of veterans, J. Missouri Med. Ass. 44:651-654, 1947.

Woolsey, R. D., and Tsang, J. L. K.: Review of 300 cases of protruded discs treated surgically, J. Int. Coll. Surg. 18:456-463, 1952.

Wycis, H. T.: Contralateral recurrent herniated disks, Arch. Surg. 60:274-278, 1950.

Yale, D. I.: A follow-up study after surgery for ruptured lumbar intervertebral discs, Guthrie Clin. Bull. 29:126-131, 1960.

Yamada, K.: The dynamics of experimental posture. Experimental study of intervertebral disc herniation in bipedal animals, Tokushima J. Exp. Med. 8:350-361, 1962; Clin. Orthop. 25:20-31, 1962.

Youmans, J. R., and Mitchell, O. C.: Diagnosis and treatment of low back pain with emphasis on the herniated disc, J. S. Carolina Med. Ass. 62:267-276, 1966.

Young, H. H.: Additional lesions simulating protruded intervertebral disc, J. Int. Coll. Surg. 17:831-839, 1952; correction 52:312, 1952.

Young, H. H.: Posterior fusion of vertebrae in treatment for protruded intervertebral disk, J. Neurosurg. 19:314-318, 1962.

Young, J. G.: Intervertebral disk disease; new syndromes and new concepts, Med. J. Aust. 2:234-245, 1945.

Young, J. H.: Recent advances in diagnosis and treatment of lumbar intervertebral disk disease, Med. J. Aust. 1:45-49, 1946.

Young, J. H.: Intervertebral disc disease; its recognition and treatment by general practitioner, New Zeal. Med. J. 47:106-114, 1948.

Young, R. H.: Protrusion of intervertebral discs, Proc. Roy. Soc. Med. 40:233-236, 1947.

Zaaijer, J. H.: Operative verification of discograms, Arch. Chir. Neerl. 5:76-80, 1953.

Zervopoulas, G.: Diagnosis and localization of herniated intervertebral disks, Neurology 6:754, 1956.

INDEX

A

Age
of lumbar disc disease patient, relation to mode of therapy, 39
of onset of leg pain, relation to disability following surgery for lumbar disc disease, 53
in predicting future disability in lumbar disc disease patient, 53, 54, 55, 56-57
relationship to disability following conservative therapy for lumbar disc disease, 54
relationship to disability following surgery for lumbar disc disease, 53

Ankle reflexes
decreased or absent, scoring in factor analysis of disability, 102
decreased, following therapy for lumbar disc disease, table, 46
"normal," relation to disability following surgery for lumbar disc disease, 53
status in lumbar disc disease, 28

Ankylosis, evaluation of, 88, 89, 91

Anterior bony fringing, frequency of findings in follow-up roentgenograms compared to reference hospital roentgenograms, 62, 63

Arthritis
hypertrophic
association with low back pain, 66
in patients with lumbar disc disease, incidence in study, 10
Marie-Strumpell, association with low back pain, 66

Articular facets
asymmetry of, discovery in roentgenographic evaluation of lumbar spine, 62, 63
changes in, association with lumbosacral disc degeneration, 65

Asymmetry of articular facets, discovery in roentgenographic evaluation of lumbar spine, 62, 63

Atrophy
of leg muscles
relation to other components of disability in lumbar disc disease, 49
scoring in factor analysis of disability, 102
following therapy for lumbar disc disease, table, 46
of muscles in lumbar disc disease, 24, 25, 32

Axis, lumbar, changes in, association with lumbosacral disc degeneration, 65

B

Back
instructions for examination, 85
manipulation of, for lumbar disc disease, 35
use of
instructions for evaluation, 86
limitation due to pain, scoring in factor analysis of disability, 103
limitation due to weakness, scoring in factor analysis of disability, 103

Back conditions in predicting future disability of lumbar disc disease patient, 53, 54, 55

Back pain
in lumbar disc disease, onset, 10-12
relationship to other components of disability in lumbar disc disease patient, 49
scoring in factor analysis of disability, 104

Bed rest for lumbar disc disease, 35

Body cast for lumbar disc disease, 35

Bony fringing
anterior, frequency of findings in follow-up roentgenograms compared to reference hospital roentgenograms, 62, 63
association with lumbosacral disc degeneration, 65, 66
posterior, frequency of findings in follow-up roentgenograms compared to reference hospital roentgenograms, 62

Brace for lumbar disc disease, 35

Bursitis in patients with lumbar disc disease, incidence in study, 10

C

Calcification of disc, frequency of findings in follow-up roentgenograms compared to reference hospital roentgenograms, 62

Calcification of intervertebral disc space, association with lumbosacral disc degeneration, 65

Calculi, urinary, in patients with lumbar disc disease, incidence in study, 10

Cast, body, for lumbar disc disease, 35

Cervical disc rupture in patients with lumbar disc disease, incidence in study, 10

Clinical history of lumbar disc disease, 10-16

Clinical signs by physical examination in lumbar disc disease, 17-33

Clinical study of lumbar herniated nucleus pulposus, implementation, 3-5